THE HEART AND CIRCULATORY SYSTEM

PROJECTS FOR YOUNG SCIENTISTS

PROJECTS FOR
YOUNG SCIENTISTS

THE HEART AND CIRCULATORY SYSTEM

BY ROBERT E.
DUNBAR

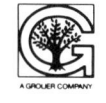

FRANKLIN WATTS
NEW YORK | LONDON | TORONTO | SYDNEY | 1984

FOR MY DAUGHTER,
YVETTE

Diagrams by Vantage Art
Illustrations by Anne Canevari Green
Photographs courtesy of
Marquette Electronics, Inc., Milwaukee, Wisconsin: p. 27;
Lafayette Instrument Company: p. 45;
Ealing Corporation, Harvard Bioscience Division: p. 47;
Collins Survey (Stead-Wells(R)—
Stead-Wells is a registered trademark of Warren E. Collins, Inc.),
Warren E. Collins, Inc.: p. 60; Autogenics/Cyborg: p. 70;
Carolina Biological Supply Company: p. 73.

Library of Congress Cataloging in Publication Data

Dunbar, Robert E.
The heart and circulatory system.

(Projects for young scientists)
Includes index.
Summary: Describes the functioning of the heart and circulatory system, presenting numerous related projects, and including information on science scholarships, grants, and awards.
1. Cardiovascular system—Experiments—Juvenile literature. (1. Circulatory system—Experiments. 2. Experiments) I. Title. II. Series.
QP103.D86 1984   612'.1   84-7382
ISBN 0-531-04766-0

Copyright © 1984 by Robert E. Dunbar
All rights reserved
Printed in the United States of America
5 4 3 2 1

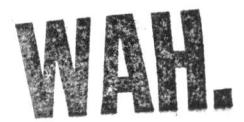

CONTENTS

CHAPTER 1
The Most Vital Organ
1

CHAPTER 2
Working Scientifically
9

CHAPTER 3
Observation Projects
13

CHAPTER 4
Demonstration Projects
35

CHAPTER 5
Construction Projects
77

CHAPTER 6
Writing a Scientific Report
87

CHAPTER 7
Preparing for
Science Competitions
91

CHAPTER 8
Prizes, Scholarships,
Grants
and Other Awards
93

APPENDIX
Sources for Equipment
and Other
Project Needs
99

INDEX
101

ACKNOWLEDGMENT

I would like to acknowledge the
generous assistance given me
by four Maine resource persons
in the writing of this book.

They are:
KENNETH A. LUTTE,
chairman of the Science Department,
Lincoln Academy, Newcastle;

PHILIP MARCOUX,
chairman of the Science Department,
Georges Valley High School, Thomaston;

DR. CHARLES E. HUNTINGTON,
chairman, and
DR. BEVERLY N. GREENSPAN,
associate professor,
Department of Biology,
Bowdoin College, Brunswick.

1
THE MOST VITAL ORGAN

Your heartbeat is so familiar and so constant that you probably give it little thought when conditions are normal. Even though you may experience a rapid heartbeat from time to time, due to physical exertion, you go about your daily business, unconcerned, though the exhaustion, shortness of breath, and rapid heartbeat may make you want to slow down and rest for a while so you can feel comfortable again.

You may experience the same kind of exhaustion when subjected to emotional stress. Although you may not feel physically tired, there may be shortness of breath and rapid heartbeat when your mind is emotionally upset. A quarrel that leads to a shouting match; a conflict with parents or friends; a poor grade that was unexpected; losing a sporting match; being turned down or rejected by someone in whom you are romantically interested—all of these situations may affect you emotionally. They may also put a temporary strain on your heart, just as physical exhaustion can. If your heart is healthy, there is no danger. When you recover physically and emotionally, your heartbeat will return to its normal rhythm.

Without a healthy heart, however, you cannot survive prolonged physical and emotional strain. Every living cell in your body and all your organs, including your brain, depend on the heart to survive and function. If any organ can be called "the vital force" that makes life possible, it is the heart.

Basically, the heart is a pump that keeps fresh blood coursing through your body, bringing oxygen and nutrients to all your organs and cells. A mathematical description of what the heart accomplishes every second of your life is astonishing. Your heart keeps approximately 10 pints (4.73 liters) of blood constantly circulating through 75,000 miles (120,000 km) of blood vessels. These blood vessels nourish about 300 trillion cells, keeping them alive and healthy so all your organs can function to keep you in good health and protected from disease. The circulating blood nourishes every cell in your body by providing oxygen and nutrients. It also carries away the carbon dioxide and other waste products that your body cannot use. This must be done without interruption if you are to remain healthy and alive.

Every living cell in your body depends on oxygen for life. Any cell deprived of oxygen for more than thirty minutes will die. The cells in your brain are even more dependent on a fresh and constant supply of oxygen. If your brain is totally deprived of oxygen for just five seconds, this will cause a blackout or unconsciousness. If your heart stops and your brain is deprived of oxygen for more than four minutes, your brain will die. "Brain death" is accepted by the medical profession as evidence of death, even though other organs may survive longer.

That's why the heartbeat is considered a "vital sign." As long as your heart keeps beating, you have a chance to continue living, no matter what illness or injury may have damaged your body. The heartbeat is physical evidence that the inside of your body is in a constant state of change. Every cell and organ must be constantly nourished; the waste products must be removed. The blood must continue to circulate, powered by that vital muscular device called the heart.

When blood flow stops, the effect in humans is first noticed in the brain and the nervous system it controls. Without a constant flow of blood to provide oxygen and nutrients and to remove waste products, its functioning quickly breaks down. Some oxygen-dependent animals, however, have simpler and less demanding nervous systems. Their nervous systems may continue to function for a relatively long time (several hours or even days or weeks) after the heart has stopped beating.

William Harvey (1578–1657) discovered that blood circulates throughout the body. He could not explain, however, the motion of the heart that makes circulation possible. As far as he was concerned, that could be "comprehended only by God." More than 300 years later, some questions still remained unanswered, although a great deal of progress has been made in understanding how the heart functions and how it is controlled.

The motion of the heart appears to be inherent in the heart itself. In one experiment, the heart of a turtle was removed from its body and kept on beating for a long time. Even small pieces of heart tissue that have been kept alive in solutions may continue to contract and relax rhythmically. The heartbeat appears to be an innate quality of the heart muscle, controlled by a complex system of electrical impulses within the heart itself.

The normal rate of heartbeat in humans is about 70 beats per minute. But the rate in other forms of life varies greatly. When a hummingbird is out searching for food, its heart rate is sometimes as high as 1,000 beats per minute. By contrast the huge and usually slow-moving elephant has a heart rate that is only 30 beats per minute. A slow heart rate is also a characteristic of animals that hibernate. The slow heartbeat helps the animal conserve the energy it has stored up in its body.

As far as heartbeat in humans is concerned, the normal rate will vary according to the physiological makeup of the person, the activity he or she is engaged in, and the needs of the body at a particular time. Sometimes your heart may beat twice as fast as normal because your body tissues need increased supplies of blood and oxygen. This can happen during exercise, when you are emotionally excited, or when you have a fever. The flow of blood must vary to meet the body's needs. The healthy heart cooperates by increasing either the volume of blood released for circulation or the number of beats per minute.

Another way in which your heartbeat is controlled is through the body's nervous system. Nerve impulses come from the spinal cord or the brain, either increasing or slowing the heart rate in the process. All your body's nervous systems are connected to the brain, which is the primary source of heart rate control. Increased pressure in the arteries also stimulates nerves; an episode of rapid beating increases the pressure, and this can tend to slow the heartbeat. In this way, your nervous system helps keep your pulse rate at a normal level when you are calm and at rest. But, as you will discover, the brain, other vital organs, and the nervous system act and interact in a much more complex way in affecting the heartbeat.

HEART, BLOOD, AND LUNGS

An adequate supply of oxygen is essential to your heartbeat as well as to the health of all the organs and cells in your body. The heart plays a crucial role in serving this need. But the heart, in turn, is dependent on the functioning of your lungs. As you breathe, your lungs take in oxygen. This is absorbed by the blood that courses from your lungs into your heart via vessels called the pulmonary veins. From the heart the oxygenated blood is sent on its way to all the organs and cells in your body. As the cells absorb oxygen and nutrients from the blood, they give off carbon dioxide and other waste products. Two large veins, the venae cavae, bring blood back to the heart from all parts of the body. This blood carries very little oxygen and a lot of carbon dioxide. From the heart, the blood is pumped through the pulmonary arteries to the lungs, where the carbon dioxide is expired from the body. The rate of respiration in humans mainly depends on how quickly oxygen is absorbed by cells and organs, and carbon dioxide expired by the lungs. This action is governed by how often and how deeply we breathe.

You might expect that the lungs have muscles, just as the heart does, to make the inspiration of oxygen and the expiration of carbon dioxide possible. But the lungs do not have muscles. They are forced to expand and allowed to relax through movements of the ribs, which form a "cage" around the lungs, and the diaphragm, a muscular organ located at the lower end of the ribs. Like your heartbeat, the rhythmic motion of your lungs in expanding and relaxing is a constant process, continuing whether you are awake or asleep. You can control your breathing to some extent. If you feel like taking a deep breath, for example, you can do so immediately. But you can't make your heart beat faster or slower on impulse.

You have the power to hold your breath or stop breathing, but not for very long. If you hold your breath long enough, you will lose consciousness and then start breathing again automatically. The reason for this is that the muscles in your ribs and diaphragm are controlled by the body's nervous system. This has been confirmed by experiments on animals. When the nerves to these muscles are severed, breathing stops and cannot be resumed. The ability to breathe can be threatened by certain diseases, among them poliomyelitis, or infantile paralysis. When the nerves that control breathing are damaged beyond repair, a person can be kept alive only by continuous artificial respiration provided by "iron lungs" or other life-supporting devices.

The rhythm of breathing is controlled by a nerve center located in the lower part of the brain. This center sends rhythmic impulses to rib and diaphragm muscles that permit the relaxation and expansion of the lungs. When you want to stop breathing, the "message" comes from the brain's breathing center which acts on the nervous system voluntarily, in other words by your "willing" it to happen. Breathing can also stop *involuntarily*, without your realizing that it has happened. For example, you automatically stop breathing when you swallow. Breathing also stops when you are frightened and quickly catch your breath or when you smell toxic fumes that irritate your nostrils or lungs.

The amount of carbon dioxide in your blood also helps to regulate your breathing. If your body's cells and organs are giving off unusually high amounts of carbon dioxide, your breathing rate will increase so you can force more carbon dioxide out and a fresh supply of oxygen in. What if an unusually low amount of carbon dioxide is absorbed by your blood on its way back to the heart and lungs? This isn't likely, but if it happens, your breathing rate will decrease.

Under normal conditions, however, the buildup of carbon dioxide in the blood acts on the breathing center in your brain, forcing you to breathe. This is how the body maintains a balance between the amount of carbon dioxide given off as waste products and the amount of oxygen needed to replace it. This balance is regulated automatically in a healthy human.

The absorption of oxygen and expiration of carbon dioxide is a continuous process that begins at birth. Its success in maintaining life depends on the most vital organ in your body, your heart.

CHALLENGE YOUR SKILLS

In the sections that follow you will find three types of projects to challenge your skills and increase your knowledge of the heart—observation projects, demonstration projects, and construction projects. Working with your instructor's guidance, either alone or with other students, you may want to enter one of these projects in a science competition to find out how your work compares with your peers as well as to compete for honors and prizes.

You will also find sections on writing a scientific report, preparing for science fairs and other competitions, and a listing of some of the national competitions that offer scholarship grants and other awards. There is also a section on sources of special equipment, animal specimens, and organs you may need to complete a project.

2

WORKING SCIENTIFICALLY

Scientists are often faced with problems or questions about the functioning of the human body. In seeking answers to questions, the scientist tries to solve a problem by forming a tentative answer, or hypothesis. The hypothesis is meaningless, however, unless it can be tested by an experiment. The scientist records what happens and can use the results to show whether the hypothesis is right or wrong.

This sequence of events is known as the scientific method. It forms the basis for all scientific research and for the projects in this book.

Whatever project you work on will have special conditions and require certain procedures. You should perform these procedures using scientific methods. This involves certain basic principles, such as reference to authority, observation, trial and error, experimental control, the need for repetition, and awareness of sources of error. Use your school library and other sources recommended by your instructor to familiarize yourself with research that relates directly to your project. This background will help to give you a good understanding of the particular problem you are dealing with and may suggest additional questions to investigate.

CONTROLLED EXPERIMENTS

For the results of a project to be scientifically valid, you must conduct controlled experiments. This means that only one factor at a time may be varied. If you were to vary two factors at the same time, it would be impossible to state definitely that the outcome of the experiment was based on one factor rather than the other.

During a project, you will change certain conditions and observe and record the results. In a controlled experiment you will work with both independent and dependent variables. When you change a factor in an experiment to observe the results, the factor that you change is known as an independent variable. When this factor causes a second factor to change, the second factor is known as the dependent variable. In other words, a variable is something that is changed (independent) or shows change (dependent) in a particular experiment.

You will conduct experiments under precisely known and noted conditions so that you can learn the effects of varying a single factor at a time. You will control your experiments to satisfy yourself that the factor varied is the only one causing any observed difference. One way to do this is to duplicate the experiment exactly except in one respect—the variable under consideration is not allowed to change. Where needed, studies may be repeated to make sure that the results do not vary significantly and that all the conditions required by the project design have been followed as exactly as possible.

PREPARATION AND PROCEDURE

Before you begin an experiment, make sure you have all of the supplies, equipment, and other materials you need. Proceed with each step of the experiment as accurately as possible according to the conditions required by the project design. Where timing is involved, it should be performed exactly as specified. Quantities of chemical substances should be measured with care. Any inaccuracies in timing or in quantities of chemical substances will invalidate your results.

The same attention to accuracy is also important in the records you keep of each procedure in an experiment and the results you obtain. All the details you record in your notebook—procedures followed, observations, and results—should be made as they happen, when they are fresh in your mind. By keeping accurate and complete notes of each project, you will be rewarded when the time comes to write your scientific report. The completeness and importance of each section of the report will depend on how thorough and accurate your notes are. You will also need them for whatever graphs and other illustrative material are needed to substantiate the accuracy and importance of your results.

3

OBSERVATION PROJECTS

STRUCTURE AND FUNCTION OF THE HEART

The heart has many components that work together in determining and controlling blood pressure and pulse rate. The heart is a four-chambered muscular organ that pumps a continuous flow of blood throughout the body's circulatory system. A normal, healthy heart will beat about 100,000 times each day and pump 1,800 gallons (7,200 liters) of blood to meet the body's needs. The heart is divided into two sides, a left and a right side. Each side has a chamber in which blood collects, called an atrium, and a chamber that pumps blood out of the heart, called a ventricle.

The heart is attached to tubes, or blood vessels, that go to all parts of the body. The blood vessels that take blood away from the heart are arteries; blood is returned to the heart along blood vessels called veins.

On the right side of the heart, the atrium receives blood on its return from the portion of the circulatory system which supplies the body cells, the venae cavae. This is blood that has been depleted of oxygen, which has been replaced with carbon dioxide and other waste products. This blood passes from the right atrium into the right ventricle, which then pumps it into the lungs along the pulmonary artery. In the lungs the carbon dioxide is eliminated through expiration and replaced with oxygen through inspiration.

The oxygen-rich blood then flows through the pulmonary vein into the atrium on the left side of the heart, passing from there to the left ventricle. From the left ventricle the fresh supply of oxygen-rich blood is pumped out of the heart along the aorta. This is the major artery that carries blood away from the heart. Blood is distributed to all parts of the body by means of the arterial system. This consists of arteries, small arteries called arterioles, and capillaries, which are the tiniest blood vessels. After supplying all the body's organs, tissues, and cells with oxygen and other nutrients, the blood carries carbon dioxide and other waste products back to the heart through the body's venous system. As part of the circulatory process, soluble waste products are removed by the kidneys and excreted. The venous system consists of veins and smaller veins called venules, which, like the arterioles, are connected to the capillaries.

The pumping action of the heart is controlled by a natural pacemaker. This is a small bundle of highly specialized muscle cells located in the upper right side of the heart. The pacemaker cells generate the electrical impulses that coordinate the contractions of the heart. The pacemaker, in turn, is controlled by the vagus nerve, which acts to slow the heart rate, and accelerator nerves, which act to increase heart rate. These actions directly affect the flow and volume of blood as well as heartbeat.

When the heart relaxes, the decrease in pressure within the heart allows blood to flow into the atria. It also allows the valves between the atria and ventricles to open. When the atria contract, the blood flows from the atria to the ventricles. Continuing the cycle, when the ventricles contract forcefully, the valves between the atria and ventricles close and blood is forced out of the heart. Blood from the right ventricle flows into the lungs to receive a fresh supply of oxygen. Blood from the left ventricle, already supplied with oxygen and other nutrients, begins its journey through the body's circulatory system, supplying the body cells. Circulation of the blood is a continuous process, without interruption or impediment in a healthy human being.

PROJECT 1:
Blood vessels of the heart

Using a book on anatomy as a reference, in the unmarked illustration of the heart provided on page 16, locate the following blood vessels of the heart: pulmonary artery, aorta, inferior vena cava, superior vena cava, pulmonary veins, and coronary vessels. Explain the function of each.

PROJECT 2:
Muscles in the heart

On the illustration provided, locate the papillary muscles in the left and right ventricles and the chorda tendinae. Using a book on anatomy as a reference, describe how these structures function in the beating heart.

PROJECT 3:
Blood flow in the heart

On the illustration provided, starting from the right atrium, trace the flow of blood through the following structures:

Right atrium	Lungs
Left atrium	Pulmonary artery
Mitral valve	Aorta
Tricuspid valve	Pulmonary semilunar valve
Right ventricle	Aorta semilunar valve
Left ventricle	Pulmonary veins

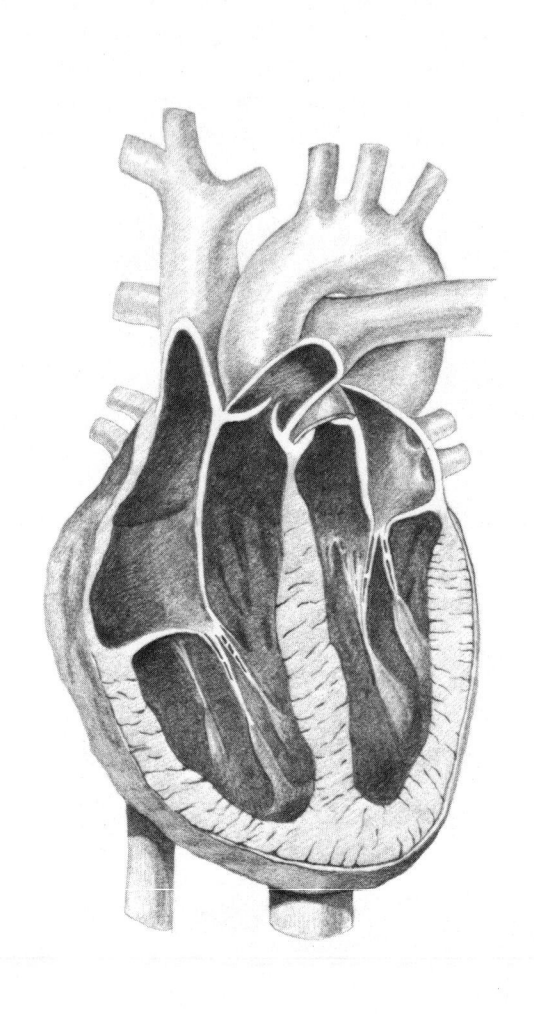

THE HUMAN HEART

CHANGES IN BLOOD PRESSURE AND PULSE RATE

When a scientist speaks of blood pressure, he or she is referring to the force that the blood exerts in all directions in a given area. Blood pressure is responsible for completing the circulatory process of the blood from the heart to all parts of the body and then back to the heart. According to principles of physics, fluids move from an area of high pressure to an area of low pressure. This is a constant process in the human body. Blood pressure at different parts of the body, however, will vary according to four factors: the amount of blood present; the size of the vessel through which the blood flows; the force of the heartbeat; and the resistance encountered to the flow of blood.

When a person is sitting or lying down, for example, the pressure along an artery will be highest at the point that is closest to the heart. When a person stands up, the force of gravity will cause the blood to collect in the lower parts of the body. Both arterial and venous pressures in the feet will be higher than they are in the head.

In assessing a person's blood pressure, two measurements are taken. One is called systolic pressure, the other diastolic pressure. The systolic pressure is higher than the diastolic. The systolic phase occurs when the ventricles of the heart contract and force blood into the arteries. When the ventricles relax, blood flows from the atria through the atrioventricular valves, the mitral and tricuspid valves, into the ventricles. The lowest point of pressure, the diastolic phase, occurs just before the ventricles contract. Keep in mind, however, that the pressure at any given point in an artery is never constant. It is always changing between high, or systolic, pressure and low, or diastolic, pressure, in response to the pumping action of the heart.

Blood pressure is measured by determining how high it will raise a column of mercury, with the results ex-

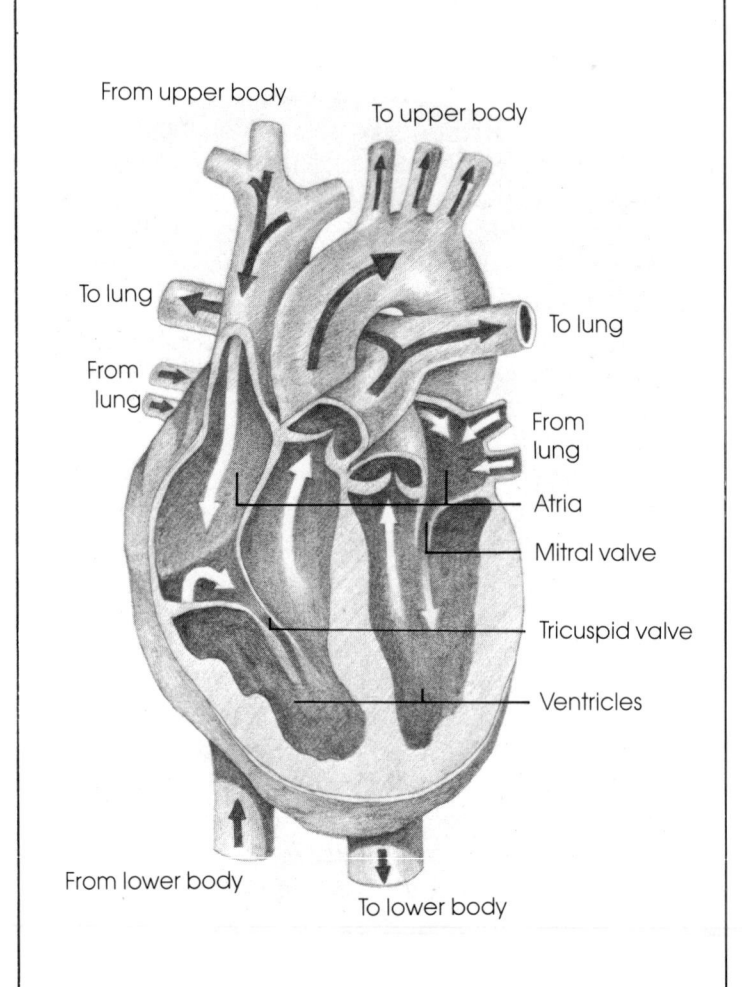

**CROSS-SECTION OF THE HEART
SHOWING ANATOMY AND BLOOD FLOW**

pressed in millimeters (mm Hg). In recording the results, the systolic pressure is written first and then the diastolic pressure. It is expressed in the following way, for example, 120/80 mm Hg. A third measurement of blood pressure is called the pulse pressure. This is a measurement of the difference between the systolic and diastolic pressures between heartbeats. In the foregoing example, the difference, or pulse, pressure is 40 mm Hg. Pulse pressure is an expression of the approximate output of the heart during ventricular systole.

TAKING BLOOD PRESSURE READINGS

The most accurate measurement of blood pressure requires the insertion of a needle directly into an artery and connecting it to a mercury manometer or electronic transducer. However, this method is not considered practical in routine examinations of blood pressure. The most familiar method involves the use of a sphygmomanometer. This device consists of an inflatable cuff, an inflation pump, a gauge to register pressure, and a controlled exhaust valve. Using the sphygmomanometer is less precise but it is considered appropriate for most blood pressure examinations. It is the method commonly used by physicians in examining patients.

First the cuff is wrapped around the subject's upper arm just above the elbow and then inflated. When the pressure in the cuff exceeds that in the artery being tested, the artery collapses and blood flow stops. Readings are taken as the pressure in the cuff is gradually released. This allows the blood to flow through the artery again. The readings taken will be keyed to the sounds that result when the blood begins to circulate again.

LISTENING FOR SOUNDS

Using a stethoscope, the sounds that are heard are known as Korotkov's sounds, and they occur in five phases. These sounds are caused by the vibration of the arterial wall and by the turbulently flowing blood as it moves through the narrowed artery into the fully opened artery below the cuff. In Phase 1, clear, tapping sounds are heard that increase in intensity as the cuff pressure decreases. The point at which the first regular tapping sound occurs during deflation of the cuff represents the highest, or systolic, pressure.

As the cuff continues to deflate gradually, Phase 1 is followed by a softer, muffled sound, or murmur. This is Phase 2. Then you will hear a less clear, but louder, tapping sound, which is Phase 3. In Phase 4 there will be a sudden change from the loud tapping of Phase 3 to a muffled, soft blowing sound. At this point, Phase 4, the lowest, or diastolic, reading is taken.

There is one more phase in the series of Korotkov's sounds, Phase 5, in which all sound disappears. Usually this is closer to the true diastolic pressure. Phase 4 is used, however, because in some subjects Korotkov's sounds never disappear completely. This is often the case after exercise or if the subject is suffering from certain diseases. Also, it is easier to distinguish between changes in sound than to recognize the disappearance of sound.

POINTERS ON TECHNIQUE

In preparing to take blood pressure readings, the subject should be relaxed and seated comfortably, with his or her forearm on a smooth surface at heart level. Set the needle of the manometer at zero, with the cuff deflated and the exhaust valve open. The artery to be tested is the brachial artery, which is located on the inside of the upper arm, just above the bend in the elbow (see illustration). Wrap the deflated cuff around the upper arm about 3 centimeters above the bend in the elbow. It should be snug but not too tight. (Note: If you are using an electronic sphygmomanometer or a cuff with a built-

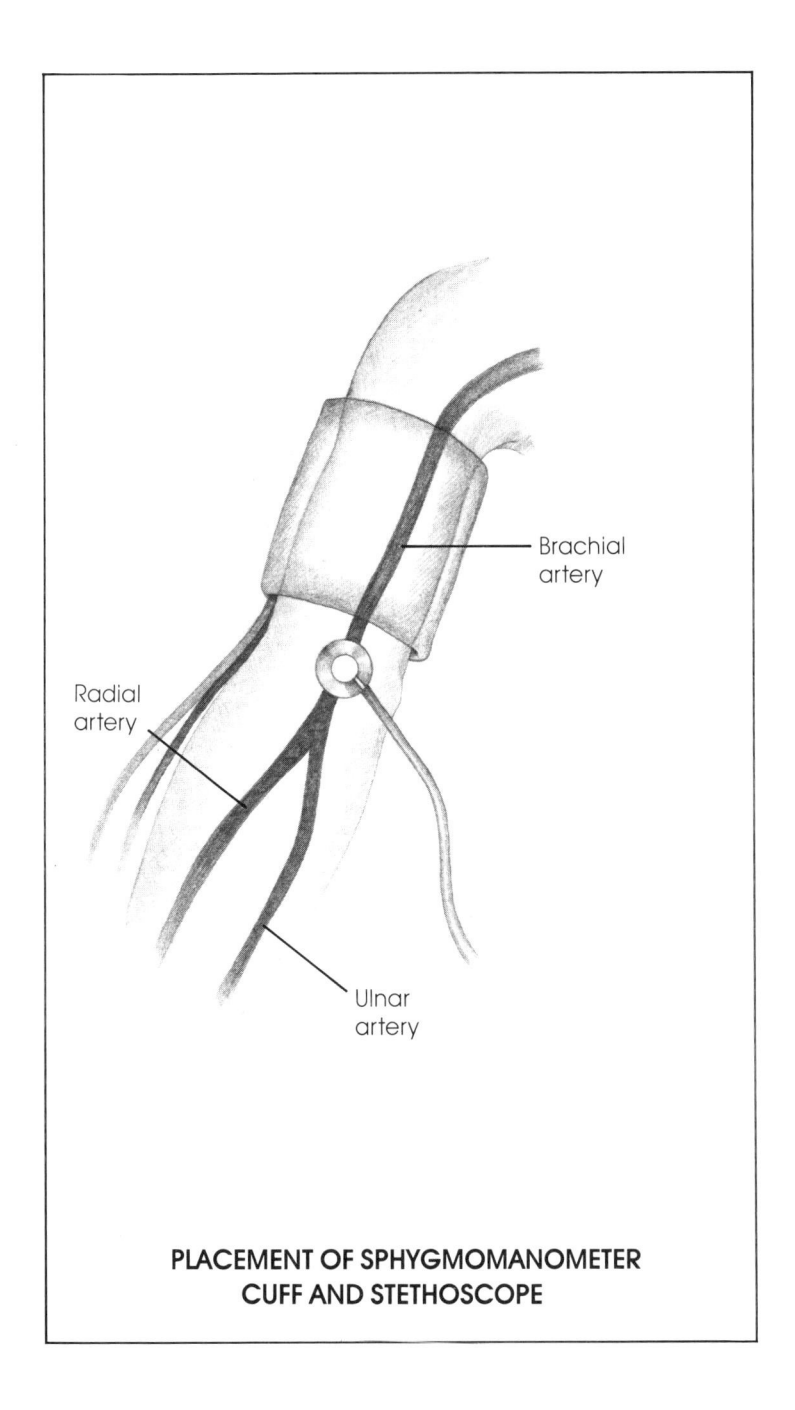

PLACEMENT OF SPHYGMOMANOMETER CUFF AND STETHOSCOPE

in stethoscope, the microphone or stethoscope bell should be directly over the brachial artery.) Use the brachial artery as a central point so that half of the inflatable bag is on either side of it.

Now use a finger to feel the pulse in the radial artery in the subject's wrist (do not use your thumb as it has its own pulse beat). At the same time, use your other hand to close the exhaust valve and inflate the cuff rapidly. The bag should be inflated to a pressure that is approximately 30 mm Hg above the point at which the pulse stops beating.

Place the stethoscope over the brachial artery just below the cuff. Open the exhaust valve and let the air out of the cuff at a rate of 2 to 5 mm Hg per second. While the air is leaving the cuff, listen closely for the first clear tapping sound (Phase 1). This will give you the reading for systolic pressure. The sounds will become muffled (Phase 2), and then you will hear a louder tapping sound (Phase 3). When the sounds become muffled for a second time, Phase 4 of Korotkov's sounds, take your reading for diastolic pressure. Then deflate the blood pressure cuff completely. *An inflated cuff should not be left on a subject's arm for more than a few seconds.*

PROJECT 4:
Lifestyle and blood pressure

Equipment and materials:
sphygmomanometer, stethoscope, stopwatch, notebook, pencil

Observe changes in pulse rate and blood pressure in a physically active young person subjected to short, intermediate, and prolonged periods of exercise. Perform the same test on a relatively inactive middle-aged person and compare the results. Interview both subjects about eating and drinking habits, recreational pursuits, the amount of sleep required, and other aspects of lifestyle that may directly affect how the heart functions. Write a summary of test results, lifestyles, and conclusions for each subject.

PROJECT 5:
Heart sounds

Equipment and materials:
stethoscope, stopwatch, notebook, pencil

In a quiet room, place your ear or a stethoscope against a subject's chest. Explore the midchest region to detect areas where heart sounds are the loudest. Describe the sounds you hear and count the number of heartbeats per minute for each area of the chest explored. Record your findings in a notebook.

PROJECT 6:
Recovering from exercise

Equipment and materials:
sphygmomanometer, stethoscope, stopwatch, notebook, pencil

Observe how the heart adjusts to exercise. Take the blood pressure and pulse rate of a subject. Then ask the subject to perform an exercise, such as jumping jacks, for one minute. Begin taking pulse rate and blood pressure readings at one-minute intervals until the subject's heart rate has returned to normal. Make notes on the subject's age, height, weight, and exercise habits before the test begins. Record the findings in your notebook.

PROJECT 7:
Arterial blood pressure

Equipment and materials:
sphygmomanometer, stethoscope, notebook, pencil

In a test for arterial blood pressure, select a subject in good health. Take the subject's pulse rate before the test begins. Use a stethoscope to listen for heart sounds above the subject's heart and in several other areas of the chest. Then, using a sphygmomanometer, take systolic and diastolic readings. Record these and other results of your test in a notebook.

PROJECT 8:
Reacting to the environment

Equipment and materials:
thermometer, sphygmomanometer, stethoscope, stopwatch, notebook, pencil

Observe how the action of the heart controls the internal environment of the body and in turn is controlled by it (feedback control). In a subject at rest in a comfortably heated room, record body temperature, pulse rate, and blood pressure. Then turn the thermostat down and open a window to make the room as cool as possible. Wait ten minutes and then record the subject's body temperature, pulse rate, and blood pressure at room temperature, noting any changes. In a third observation, ask the subject to perform exercises for five minutes in the cooled room. Note how this affects his or her body temperature, pulse rate, and blood pressure.

ELECTRICAL ACTIVITY OF THE HEART

The importance of electrical forces in the universe and in the world around us extends to all living things, including human beings and the human heart. All living tissues and organs, in fact, show evidence of an electrical field that can change suddenly during activity. The human heart is a good example of this. Each time the heart beats, cardiac muscle generates an electrical field. The electrical currents spread out over the entire body. The voltage generated by the heart is small and is equivalent to only

2 or 3 millivolts. This voltage can be measured through electrodes held in the hand or attached to the feet. Because the voltage is so low, a very sensitive oscillograph and a string galvanometer are needed to record it. These are two of the essential elements in the electrocardiograph machine, which is used to record the rate of heartbeat and the electrical activity of the heart.

The electrocardiogram provides a permanent record of the electrical variations that precede and accompany heartbeat. The events of each cardiac cycle are recorded on a special paper in a series of waves or deflections of the galvanometer. The deflections are designated by the letters P, Q, R, S, and T (see illustration on page 26).

The P wave is associated with activity of the atria. A brief fraction of a second after contraction begins, the P wave begins and then ends before the beat of the atria ceases. This indicates that when the atria contract they become electrically negative to the ventricles. All the other positive and negative waves in the electrocardiogram are related to activity of the ventricles. The first to appear is the Q wave. This is immediately followed by the R spike, which is the most prominent of all the waves.

The R spike shows up on the electrocardiogram a brief fraction of a second before the systole phase of the ventricles. It subsides as the pressure within the ventricles increases. The R spike shows the electrical impulse that causes the ventricular muscle to contract. As blood is ejected from the ventricles, the T wave appears. The shape of the T wave is variable and is sometimes inverted. One of its most valuable uses is in the detection of certain heart diseases.

USING THE ELECTROCARDIOGRAPH

An electrocardiograph should be used in a quiet room where the subject can lie down. It should be positioned away from any electrical equipment or wiring that would

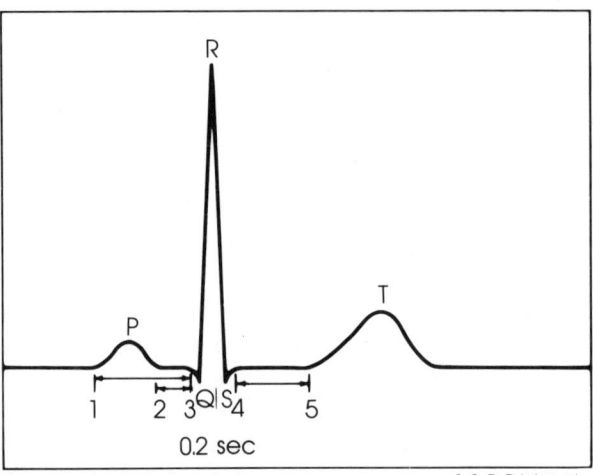

P wave – depolarization of atria
QRS complex – depolarization of ventricles
T wave – repolarization of ventricles

1-3 P-R interval
2-3 R-R segment
4-5 S-T segment

Portion of an electrocardiogram

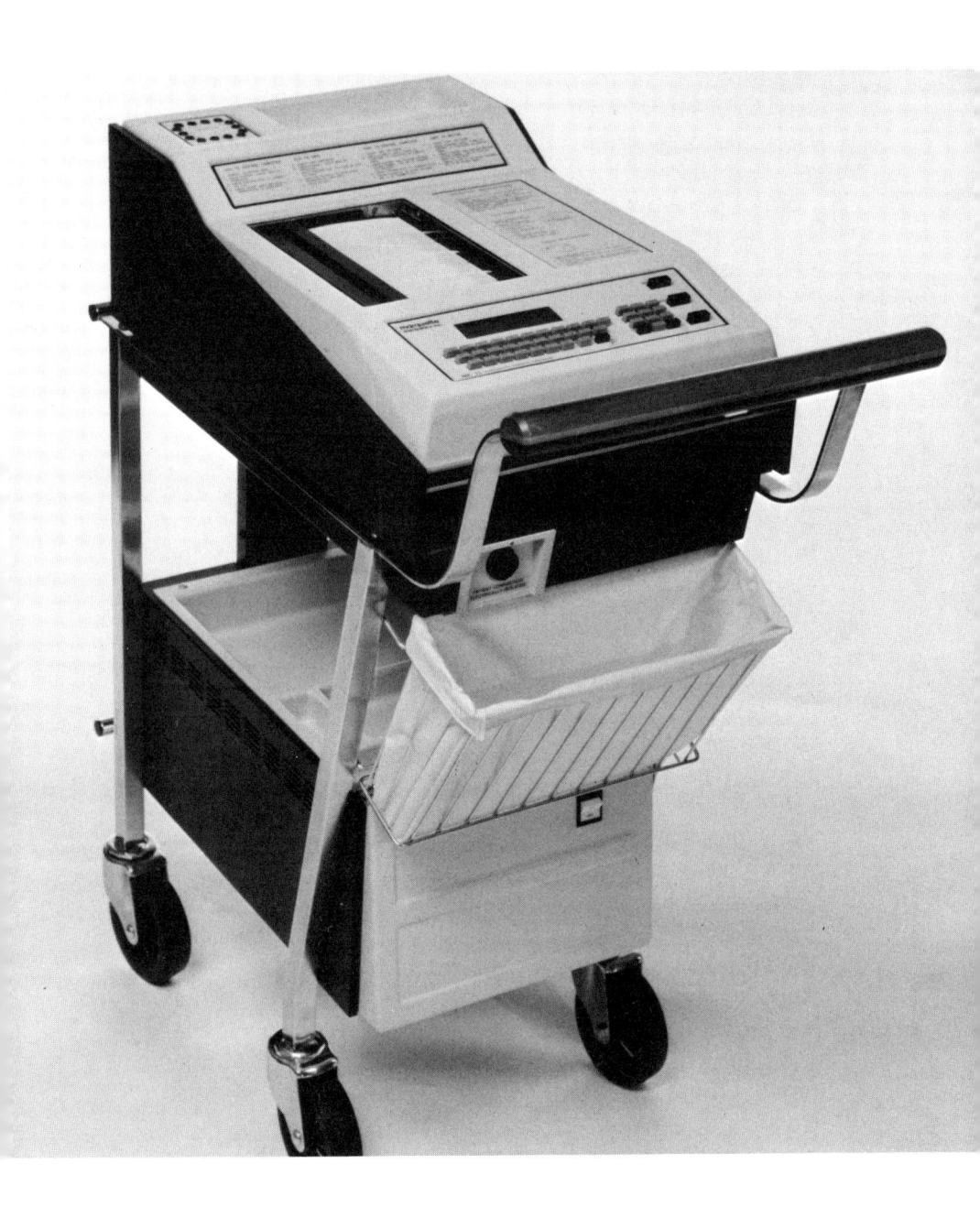

AN ELECTROCARDIOGRAPH

interfere with the recording. You should be sure you know how to operate the machine before you begin a project (see photograph on page 27).

The subject for your project should be lying down comfortably before you attach the electrodes. Make sure he or she is not in contact with any metal on the cot or nearby table. As a further precaution to prevent shock to the subject and assure the accuracy of the electrocardiogram, never touch the subject and the electrocardiograph, or any other electrical equipment, at the same time.

The electrodes should be attached to the subject with care. The electrocardiograph will not produce a reliable measurement unless good contact is made. First wash and dry the skin of the subject in the areas where the electrodes will be attached. Also wash and dry the electrodes. Rub the electrode jelly into the subject's skin at the sites where the electrodes will be attached until the skin becomes slightly red. You might want to use a tongue depressor for this part of the procedure.

Attach the rubber electrode straps to the plate electrodes by pushing the metal post on the electrode through the holes near the end of the strap. Then apply some electrode jelly to the concave surface of the electrode. Place the electrode on one of the reddened areas on the skin that you have prepared for testing. To be certain it makes good contact, rub the electrode on the skin and hold it in place by putting the rubber strap around the subject's wrist or leg. Insert the metal post of the electrode through another strap hole. Take care that it is not too loose. You don't want the electrode to slip. Neither should it be so tight that the subject is uncomfortable. Both of these conditions may interfere with the electrocardiograph recording.

After you have attached electrodes to the other sites selected, the next step is to connect cable leads to the electrodes. The RA lead, which is white, should be attached to the right-arm electrode. The black LA lead should be attached to the left-arm electrode; the RL lead, which is green, to the right-leg electrode; and the LL lead, which is red, to the left-leg electrode, etc. Before you begin taking the electrocardiogram, make sure the electrode screws are tight on the cable tips.

Now turn the lead selector switch to the STD position, and set the speed switch so that the paper will advance at 25 mm/second. Adjust the stylus heat control so that the baseline will be about 1 mm in width and black enough to be read easily. Turn the lead selector switch again so it is positioned between STD and I. You are now ready to begin recording the electrocardiogram.

Several different types of arrangements, called leads, are used to obtain electrocardiograms. Among the most common are leads I, II, and III. In lead I the electrodes are attached to the left and right wrists. In lead II the electrodes are attached to the left leg and right wrist. The electrodes in lead III are attached to the left wrist and left leg. Many other arrangements, or leads, can be used, depending on the sites selected for the test.

Moving the lead selector switch to position I, record a few heartbeats. Now advance the lead selector switch to the standby position between positions I and II on the dial. Hold it there briefly. With the dial in the standby position, press the marker button. When this is done, the marker stylus will record a dot on the recording paper. This dot will be useful later when you analyze the electrocardiogram, because it indicates that a switch to another lead was made.

Now move the lead selector switch to position II, recording several cardiac cycles before moving on to position III and any others you have selected for your project. Before you move on to each new position, be sure to hold the switch briefly in the standby position between lead settings and press the marker button.

When you have completed the electrocardiogram, move the lead selector switch to the next standby position and turn the machine off by moving the off-ground switch to the off position. The cable should then be disconnected from the machine and the electrodes removed from your subject. The subject's skin and the electrodes should be washed with soap and water and dried.

ANALYZING YOUR ELECTROCARDIOGRAM

In analyzing your electrocardiogram, compare it to examples you have at hand of normal and abnormal readings (see illustration on page 31). Identify the P wave, the QRS complex, and the T wave in your recording and make notes based on the following results.

1. Examine one section of the recording and count the number of P waves and the time interval in which they were made. You can use this information to calculate the rate per minute at which the atria beat.
2. Using the same technique, count the QRS complexes on one section of the recording and note the length of time over which they occurred. Use this information to calculate the ventricular rate per minute.
3. Describe the shape of the P wave. Is it rounded, flattened, or peaked?
4. Make a measurement of the P-R interval and note its duration in seconds. Do the same for the P-R segment. Then determine the amount of time required for the QRS complex.
5. Study the T wave variations in the leads you have selected. For example, in leads I and II is it

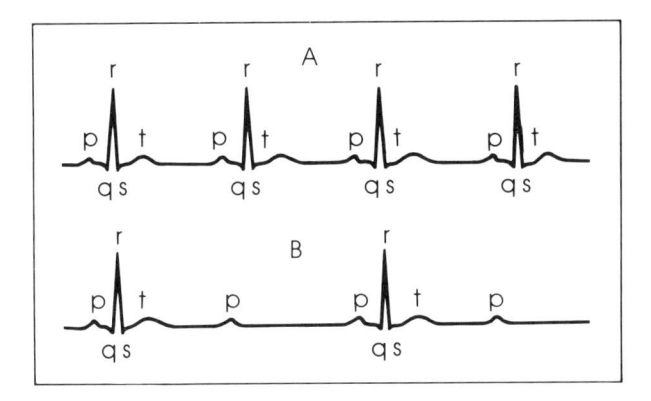

Diagram of an
Electrocardiogram.
A, normal; B, 2-1 heart block,
i.e., two auricular beats for
every ventricular beat.

positive (i.e., above the baseline of the recording)?
6. Study the S-T segment of the recording to see if it is approximately level with the P-R segment.
7. Now measure the distance between the P waves in several segments of the recording. Is the distance between the waves the same in all parts of the recording? Or does it show evidence of a sinus arrhythmia? (Note: The area of the heart that normally generates the rhythm or contractions of the heart is called the sinus node. A normal sinus rhythm indicates that the rhythm and rate of the entire heart is normal. Changes from the normal sinus rhythm are called arrhythmias.)

PROJECT 9:
Electrocardiograms and exercise

Equipment and materials:
electrocardiograph, electrode jelly, tongue depressors, notebook, pencil

Chart the passage of electrical impulses through the muscles of the heart in a subject at rest and in a subject after exercise. Note and comment on the differences revealed.

PROJECT 10:
Smoking and the heart

Equipment and materials:
electrocardiograph, electrode jelly, tongue depressors, notebook, pencil

For this project use a young adult in good health (not a student) who smokes cigarettes, a pipe, or cigars. Ask the subject not to smoke for one hour before you record the electrocardiogram. Make the recording and record the results. Now ask your subject to smoke during a ten-minute period and then make another electrocardiogram recording. In the results obtained, note any changes that can be attributed to the effects of smoking on heartbeat and electrical activity. What conclusions can you make from the results of this test?

4

DEMONSTRATION PROJECTS

PROJECT 1:
Different heart structures

Equipment and materials:
untrimmed sheep heart, scalpel, dissecting tray, blunt probe, notebook, pencil

Demonstrate your knowledge of the mammalian heart by using an untrimmed sheep heart obtained from a local butcher, slaughterhouse, or biological supply house. Place the sheep heart on a dissecting pan. The heart is covered by a membraneous sac called the pericardium. Note the number of tissue layers and also the space between the membranes of the sac. This is the pericardial cavity. Expose the heart by carefully removing the loose pericardial sac and the fat that lies above it. One recommended technique is to pull the loose pericardium forward, then dissect away from the heart. When you expose the heart, be sure to leave the associated blood vessels intact.

Note the musculature that makes up the walls of the right and left atria and ventricles. The atria are collapsed chambers and appear as small caps on either side of the heart. The ventricles take up a much larger proportion of the heart. To determine the left and right sides of the heart, note that the apex, or tapered end, of the heart points slightly to the left. Also the front surface is usually more convex than the back surface.

The pulmonary artery is a thick-walled vessel that exits from the right ventricle. This is the most conspicuous blood vessel on the front surface of the heart and branches just in front of the heart. The aorta is also a thick-walled vessel and is located behind the pulmonary artery. As it leaves the left ventricle, it ascends in front of the heart and bends to the left. Both the pulmonary artery and the aorta are connected by the ligamentum arteriosus.

Just behind the middle of the heart you will find the inferior vena cava, the great vein that carries blood to the right atrium from the lower regions of the body. The superior vena cava is the other great vein that leads into the right atrium, carrying blood from the upper portion of the body. The four pulmonary veins carry blood from the lungs to the left atrium.

Examine the interventricular groove on the back side of the heart and find the coronary vessels. This system of arteries and veins supplies the heart tissues with blood. Confirm all the above identifications with your instructor before proceeding.

Place the heart in the dissecting tray so that the front surface is facing you. Now make a lateral longitudinal incision down the length of the heart so that you have cut through the side wall of the right atrium and right ventricle. Cut only deep enough to open both chambers to view (use the accompanying illustrations as a guide). Note the tricuspid valve that separates the right atrium and ventricle. Cutting into the pulmonary artery from above, find the semilunar valve that prevents blood from flowing back into the right ventricle.

Making a similar incision on the left side of the heart, note the mitral or bicuspid valve between the left atrium and ventricle. Cut into the aorta from above to locate the aortic semilunar valve. This valve can also be found by probing into the left ventricle. Now find the papillary muscles in the left and right ventricles and the chorda tendinae which are attached to the papillary muscles and the atrioventricular valves.

Once you have identified all of the above components, you should have a clearer understanding of how blood flows into and out of the mammalian heart. To complete your demonstration, study the heart structure of birds and insects as seen in laboratory specimens. Note and discuss the similarities and differences. Explain the functions of any differences you note.

PROJECT 2:
The heart's role in
oxygen–carbon dioxide exchange

Equipment and materials:
sphygmomanometer, stethoscope, stopwatch, paper bag, notebook, pencil

Select a subject in good health. Begin the project by recording your subject's pulse rate and blood pressure. Then ask the subject to breathe very deeply for one or two minutes with his or her mouth open. Suggest a breathing rate of about fifteen breaths per minute. The subject should be told not to hurry, and the breathing should be as deep as possible. Note that it becomes increasingly more difficult to breathe deeply. The subject will probably have to make a great effort to keep going. Explain why this is so.

The subject will probably start to feel dizzy. This can be explained by the body's response to overventilation of the lungs. During overventilation the lungs wash much of the carbon dioxide out of the blood. Among other effects, this results in a fall in blood pressure. Also the blood vessels in the brain become constricted due to less than normal cerebral circulation. Record the changes in your subject's pulse rate and blood pressure. Explain these and other responses to the diminished carbon dioxide content of the blood. Does forced ventilation of the lungs have any value for a normal resting person? Explain.

In a variation of this project, ask your subject to place a paper bag over the mouth and nose, and repeat the preceding steps. Does it make it easier for your subject to continue to breathe deeply for a longer period? Why?

Ask your subject to rest for about five minutes, breathing quietly. Then ask her to pinch her nose shut and hold her breath for as long as possible. Repeat this experiment three times, each time asking your subject to ventilate her lungs thoroughly. Calculate the average length of time her breath can be held without breathing. Repeat this experiment, but first ask your subject to breathe for one minute from a paper bag before trying to hold her breath. Why are the results different?

In a third variation, ask the subject to run in place for two minutes and note how long she can hold her breath. Ask the subject to rest for five minutes and then repeat the test. Comment on the differences in the three sets of results.

VALSALVA'S EXPERIMENT

The influence of respiration on blood circulation can also be demonstrated by Valsalva's experiment. First note your subject's pulse and blood pressure. Ask your subject to inspire as fully as possible, then close her mouth immediately and hold the air in her lungs. This should be followed by a strong and prolonged effort to expire air from her lungs with the mouth remaining closed. This should cause the veins on her face and neck to become cyanotic, or bluish colored. Also note the changes in the subject's pulse rate and blood pressure. Explain these changes.

After your subject has been breathing quietly for two minutes, ask her to take a deep breath and hold it. Does this create an urge for inspiration or expiration? Have the subject repeat the test, but this time ask her to exhale deeply and not inhale for as long as possible. Explain the effect this has on the vagus nerve. What effect does this have on the heart and the oxygen–carbon dioxide exchange in the blood?

PROJECT 3:
Pollution and oxygen consumption

Equipment and materials:
One small laboratory animal (e.g., rat, guinea pig, mouse), animal chamber, rubber tube, T-tube apparatus, sodium hydroxide or soda lime, manometer, syringe, thermometer, barometer, air source such as an air pump, stopwatch, notebook, pencil

This project requires the use of a rat, guinea pig, or some other small laboratory animal. Weigh the animal to the nearest gram. Place it in an animal chamber above a supply of sodium hydroxide or soda lime and close the lid tightly (see illustration on page 40). The sodium hydroxide (or soda lime) absorbs the carbon dioxide expired by the animal. Insert a rubber tube through the chamber top and flush the chamber with a gentle stream of air for a minimum of thirty seconds. This should be done without the manometer and T-tube in place. Adjust the rubber tubing so that it reaches deeply into the chamber.

Now remove the rubber tube. With the T-tube open, insert the rubber stopper, making sure the manometer connection is held firmly in the hole in the chamber lid. You can check whether there are any leaks in the system by closing the T-tube and reducing the pressure by gently pulling back on the plunger of the syringe. Note the

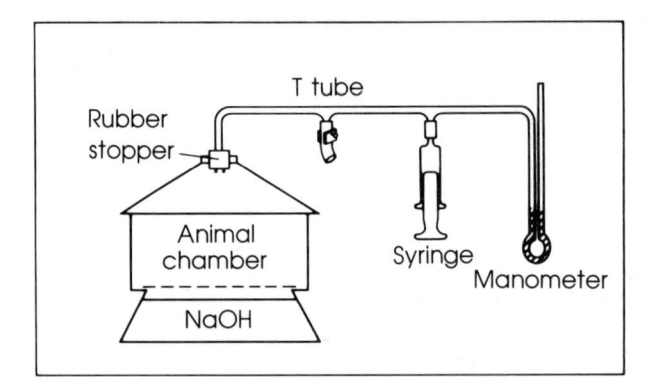

Apparatus for the measurement of oxygen consumption by small mammals

movement in the manometer fluid. Hold the syringe plunger in a fixed position for at least one minute. If the fluid level in the manometer remains constant, there is no leak in the system. Now release the syringe plunger, allowing the fluid level in both arms of the manometer to return to the same level.

Wait five minutes and then gently pull the syringe plunger back to the 50-milliliter mark, leaving the T-tube open as you do so. Then close the T-tube and make note of the time. This is called zero time (your starting time). Keep the two arms of the manometer fluid at the same level by delivering a sufficient amount of air from the syringe. Make five observations at two-minute intervals (the total time will be ten minutes), reading and recording the volume of air delivered by the syringe. Also record the temperature and barometric pressure.

When you have completed this procedure, open the clamp on the T-tube and remove the rubber stopper that holds the manometer. Flush the chamber with air. Replace the manometer and repeat the measurement of air consumption. Then repeat these procedures once more so that you will have three readings.

You can determine the metabolic rate by noting the air consumed in the last six-minute period of each run, calculating the average of the three determinations. The air volume consumed is expressed in milliliters. By dividing the volume consumed in the time period by minutes, your answer will be expressed in milliliters of air consumed per minute by the laboratory animal (ml O_2/min).

The amount of air consumed bears a direct relationship to the size of the animal. Divide the milliliters of air per minute by the mass of the animal in grams. Multiplying by 100, your answer is expressed as milliliters of air consumed per minute per 100 grams (ml O_2/min/100 g).

The heat produced by the animal can also be calculated. For each milliliter of air consumed, it has been determined that 4.8 gram calories of heat are produced.

Calculate the heat produced by multiplying the volume of air consumed by 4.8. This will give you the number of gram calories of heat produced by the laboratory animal per minute.

To record the effects of pollution on the amount of air consumed, the animal chamber is flushed with polluted air. After the animal has been placed in the chamber, insert a rubber tube through the chamber top and flush the chamber with a gentle stream of air for fifteen seconds. Then introduce polluted air (a mixture of air and sulfur dioxide or some other common pollutant such as carbon monoxide) for an additional fifteen seconds. Use an air mixture containing 5% of the pollutant. This should be done without the manometer and T-tube in place and the rubber tubing should reach deep into the chamber. Then repeat the procedure for determining air consumption. Note any changes in the behavior of the animal as well as in the amount of air consumed.

PROJECT 4:
The effect of chemicals on the heart

Equipment and materials:
fresh frog's heart, Ringer's solution, petri dish, four 250-ml beakers, blunt probe, 100 ml each of the following solutions: 0.7% sodium chloride, 0.9% potassium chloride, 1% calcium chloride, chemical additives, small fishhook, stopwatch, notebook, pencil

This project studies the effect of salts on a frog's heart that has been removed from its body. (Note: The freshly removed heart of any other laboratory specimen may also be used. It may be possible to obtain a freshly removed mammalian heart, such as beef, pig, or sheep, from a nearby slaughterhouse.) If treated with the proper mixture of salts or Ringer's solution, the frog's heart will continue to beat for an indefinite period of time. Place the heart in a petri dish of Ringer's solution and wash out the blood from the chambers by tapping the heart gently with a blunt instrument. The heart's built-in pacemaker should make it continue to beat. However if the heartbeat should stop, continue to tap the heart gently until the beating resumes.

Select four large beakers and fill each one with one of the following solutions: 0.7% sodium chloride, 0.9% potassium chloride, 1% calcium chloride solution, and Ringer's solution. Pass a fishhook through the tip of the frog's heart and tie one end of a 3-inch (7.6-cm) thread to the fishhook. The other end of the thread should be attached to the center of a pencil. Now suspend the heart in the beaker containing Ringer's solution. Count the number of beats per minute and record the result in your notebook.

Transfer the heart to the beaker containing 0.7% sodium chloride solution and repeat the procedure, counting and recording the number of beats per minute. Transfer the heart back to the Ringer's solution beaker and again count the number of beats per minute. Now transfer the heart to the beaker containing 0.9% potassium chloride solution. Count and record the number of heartbeats per minute. (Note: During this step in the procedure the heart may stop beating.)

Transfer the heart to the beaker containing 1% calcium chloride solution, counting and recording the beats per minute. This should restore the heartbeat. In the final step, transfer the heart back to the beaker containing Ringer's solution. Count and record the number of beats per minute. (Note: The heart should now be beating normally again.)

Obtain samples of chemical additives or preservatives that are commonly used in food products. Prepare several solutions, dissolving the chemicals in water. Check the percentage of additive or preservative commonly used in food products and reduce it by 10% (e.g., if the percentage is .001, reduce it to .0001). Repeat the steps in the foregoing procedure, substituting chemical additive or preservative solutions for the salt solutions. Count and record the number of heartbeats per minute. As the last step in this experiment, immerse the heart in distilled water as a control. Count and record the number of heartbeats per minute. What conclusions do you draw from the results of these tests?

PROJECT 5:
The effect of drugs on the heart

Equipment and materials:
turtle heart, kymograph or recorder with accessories—heart/smooth muscle module, wooden stylus, event/time marker module, thread, pin, heart lever, right angle clamp; turtle board, eyedropper, syringe, stopwatch, notebook, pencil; 25 ml of each of the following solutions: 1% acetylcholine, 1% adrenaline, 0.5% atropine sulfate, 10^{-5} M d-tubocurarine chloride

Either a recorder or a kymograph with accessories may be used in this project. When using a recorder (see photograph) a heart/smooth muscle module should be attached to it along with a wooden stylus to which the heart will be tied. You will also need an event/time marker module. As you begin the ink flow in the capillary pens of both modules, note that the capillary pen on the heart/smooth muscle module is counterweighted by a screw located near the ink bottle. Make sure the pen does not ride too heavily on the paper. This may interfere with the recording of heartbeats. However, the pen must make enough contact with the paper to record a line.

SMALL-ANIMAL
RECORDING SYSTEM

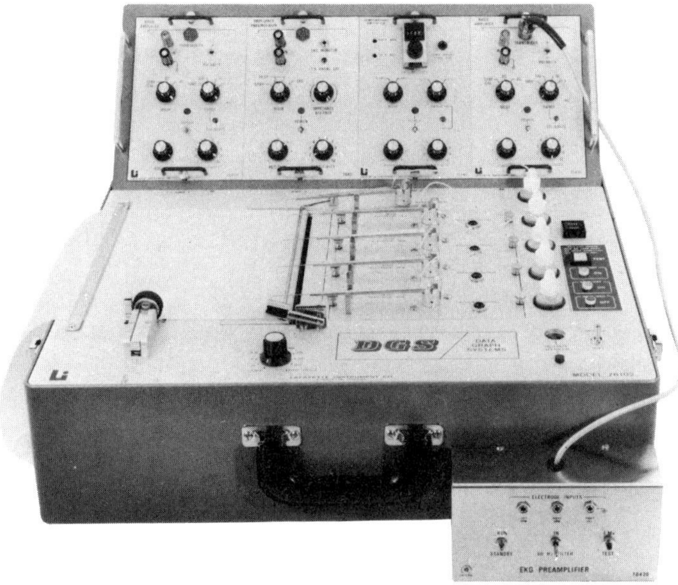
DGS
DATA GRAPH SYSTEMS
EKG PREAMPLIFIER
STANDBY
TEST

You can regulate the contact by adjusting the screw. To decrease the friction of pen against paper, turn the screw in a counterclockwise direction. The pressure of pen on paper can be increased by turning the screw in a clockwise direction.

When using a kymograph, a right angle clamp should be attached to a support stand. Insert a heart lever in the clamp with either an aluminum or wooden stylus attached to it (see photograph). Take care that the recording tip of the stylus is placed in contact with the paper on the kymograph drum. The amount of pressure exerted by the stylus against the paper must be strong enough for a mark to be made on the paper, but it should not be excessive. Excessive pressure will cause problems in recording heartbeats.

The heart of the specimen selected for your project should be tied with a piece of thread to the end of the stylus. The heart should be positioned below the stylus so that its contractions will lift the recording end of the stylus. (Note: For experiments in which electrical stimuli are applied to the vagus nerve, another right angle clamp should be attached to the support stand, positioned just below the heart level clamp.) Insert a signal magnet in the clamp, making sure its recording tip is in contact with the kymograph paper. The point of contact should be directly below the point where the heart lever stylus contacts the paper.

A turtle is recommended for this project because its heart is hardier than a frog's heart, although the heart of a large frog may be used. In the following discussion, however, we will assume that a turtle is being used.

Once the turtle has been dissected and mounted on

KYMOGRAPH WITH
ACCESSORIES

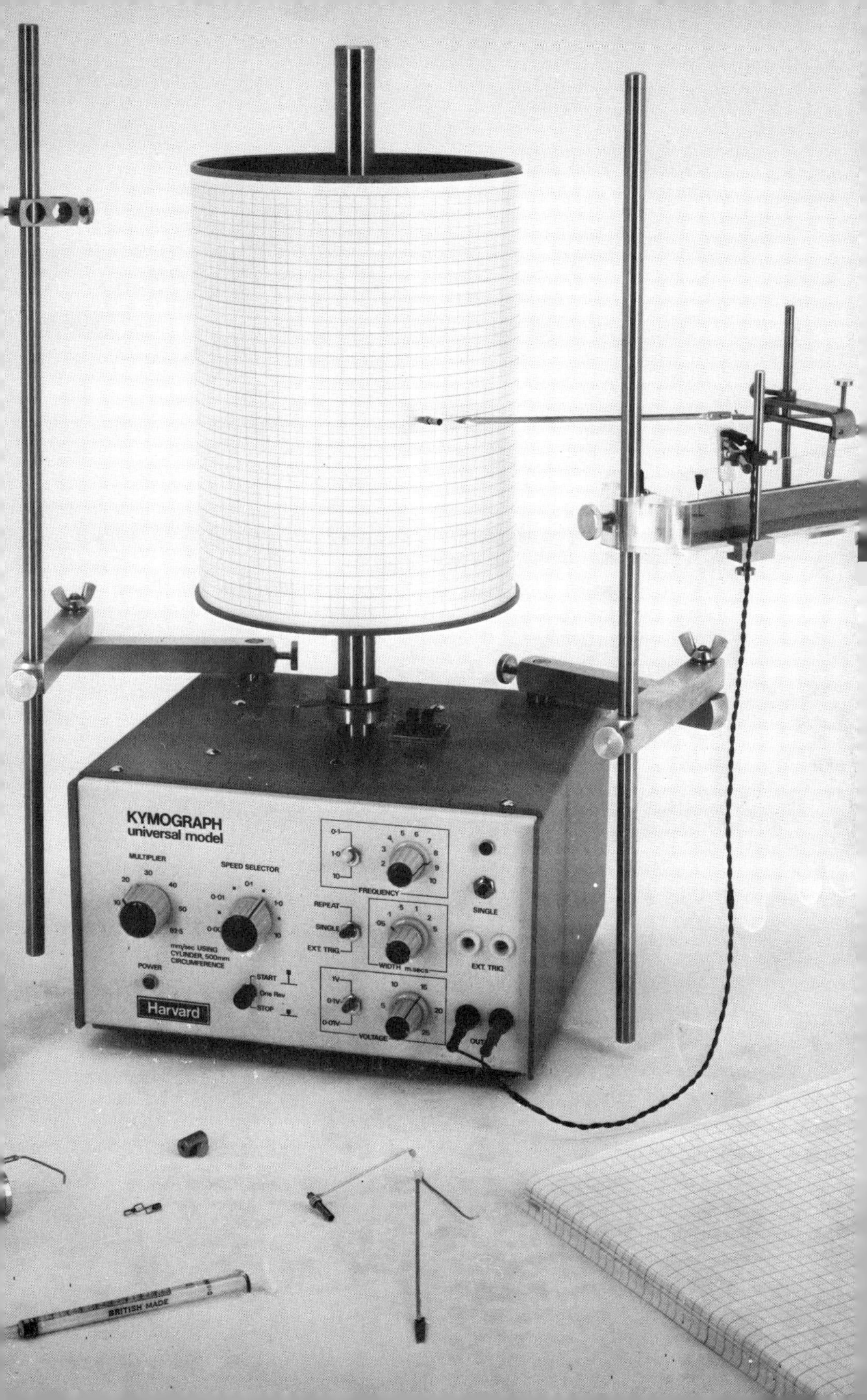
KYMOGRAPH
universal model
MULTIPLIER
SPEED SELECTOR
mm/sec USING
CYLINDER, 500mm
CIRCUMFERENCE
POWER
START
One Rev
STOP
Harvard
FREQUENCY
REPEAT
SINGLE
EXT. TRIG.
WIDTH m.secs
VOLTAGE
SINGLE
EXT. TRIG.
BRITISH MADE

a turtle board with its head exposed, a small amount of Ringer's solution should be applied to the exposed tissues. The pericardium should be slit carefully so that the heart muscle and attached blood vessels are not cut or damaged. A small bit of tissue called the frenulum anchors the apex, or pointed end, of the heart. Take an insect pin and bend it. Then tie a thread around the head of the pin and insert the tip through the frenulum. The frenulum should be cut at the end away from the heart so that the apex can be lifted. The heart should be lifted so that it is almost vertical, with the apex in the upward position. The other end of the thread should be tied to the heart lever stylus.

Note: When using the heart/smooth muscle module, the capillary pen should be deflected upward on the recorder paper each time the heart contracts. If the pen moves downward instead of upward, the heart is attached to the wrong end of the stylus.

When the heart is relaxed, the heart lever stylus should be horizontal. To make this possible, it may be necessary to attach a counterweight to the stylus at the end opposite the heart. You may want to use a small piece of modeling clay as a counterweight. This can be attached directly to the stylus. If the capillary pen moves up and down only slightly, you may need to amplify the recording. Attach the thread lifting the heart to a point that is closer to the lever's fulcrum. You can also amplify the recording by using a heavier counterweight. Take care not to stretch the heart excessively because this could prevent movement of the lever.

Turn on the paper advance mechanism of the recorder or kymograph and record several normal beats of the heart. The paper speed should be adjusted so that the peaks of ventricular contraction are recorded at approximately 2-cm intervals. This speed will enable you to detect separate atrial and ventricular beats on the recording. The atrial and ventricular contractions on the recording should be labeled as completely as possible, making note of all the experimental conditions. Note the heart rate by counting the number of contractions in a one-minute period.

Keep the heart and other exposed tissues moist with Ringer's solution, checking to make sure the heartbeat is strong and looks normal. Then run two drops of 1% acetylcholine solution onto the heart, using an eyedropper or syringe, and record the results. Wait until you notice a change in the heartbeat, and then make another recording. If no change occurs, add two or three more drops of acetylcholine solution. Note any changes in heart rate and the amplitude and duration of contractions. How long does it take for the heartbeat to recover? Wash the heart and exposed tissues with fresh Ringer's solution and proceed with the next phase of the experiment.

Make another recording and then add two drops of 1% adrenaline solution. Note the effect this has on heartbeat, recording the result. Now add two drops of 1% acetylcholine and record the result. Does the effect of adrenaline last longer than that of acetylcholine? Wash the heart and other exposed tissue with Ringer's solution until you observe that normal heartbeat has been restored.

In the next phase of the experiment, add five drops of 0.5% atropine sulfate solution and record the results. Note any changes. You should now add two or three drops of 1% acetylcholine and make a recording lasting at least one minute. What effect has the atropine solution produced? Note any changes in vagus nerve stimulation. How do the atropine effects compare with the results obtained by the other chemicals?

In the final phase of this experiment, again wash the heart and other exposed tissue with Ringer's solution and try blocking the effects of acetylcholine by adding two drops of 10^{-5}M d-tubocurarine chloride solution. How do these results compare with those obtained with atropine sulfate? What are the differences? Record all your results and conclusions in a notebook for each phase of the experiment.

HIGH BLOOD PRESSURE

Diseases of the heart and blood vessels affect an estimated twenty-nine million Americans and are the leading cause of death in the United States. The most common problem affecting the cardiovascular system is high blood pressure, also known as arterial hypertension. In most cases of hypertension there is no single, clear-cut cause; but the problem is often associated with diet, lifestyle, and inherited factors. Unfortunately, it is estimated that only about half of those who have hypertension are aware of the problem. Those who are being treated must undergo a long-term therapy that will probably involve diet, exercise, controls of other living habits, and medication. If the condition is not diagnosed and treated in time, it may lead to such coronary diseases as angina pectoris, heart attacks, strokes, and failure of other vital organs when blood vessels become damaged.

There are three factors that directly affect blood pressure: peripheral resistance, stroke volume, and heart rate. Vasoconstriction, or narrowing of the arterioles, creates peripheral resistance. As this resistance increases, the flow of blood is limited, causing an increase in blood pressure. One of the simplest demonstrations of this effect is when someone who has been lying down stands up. The arterioles narrow, increasing peripheral resistance to maintain a constant pressure and flow of blood to the brain. The response is different, however, when a person is undergoing strenuous exercise. Under these circumstances the arterioles widen to allow a more rapid flow of blood to the skeletal muscles. This is one of the benefits of exercise.

Stroke volume is the volume of blood ejected from the left ventricle during each systole. This will mainly depend on the amount of blood that fills the heart. When the ventricle pumps out a larger than normal volume of blood in one stroke, the systolic pressure will be higher. When the heart muscle is stretched in response to the larger volume of blood, it will contract more forcibly.

Under normal conditions the ventricle will pump out all the blood it contains. Therefore, any factors that tend to increase the volume of blood expelled by the ventricle will also increase systolic pressure. During exercise, for example, the return of blood to the heart will be increased by activity of the skeletal muscles and deep breathing, which stimulates the circulatory system.

Heart rate alone can also affect blood pressure. When the heart rate increases, this allows for less "runoff" time. This tends to increase the blood pressure. Blood pressure may also be increased when the heart rate is extremely low. The slowness of the heart rate allows more time for the ventricle to fill with blood. It is not unusual for athletes in training to exhibit a slow heart rate and a high systolic pressure.

PROJECT 6:
The heart's response to standing still

Equipment and materials:
sphygmomanometer, stethoscope, notebook, pencils, graph paper, stopwatch

For this demonstration you will need two subjects and an assistant to help you collect data. Select subjects of different age and sex. Ask the first subject to lie down and rest quietly for a few minutes. When the subject is completely relaxed, take his or her heart rate and blood pressure and record the data in your notebook.

Ask the subject to stand against a wall as quietly as

possible for about fifteen minutes. During this time interval, record the subject's blood pressure and heart rate simultaneously every two minutes (an assistant is needed so this can be done at the same time). Ask the subject not to move, contract his or her leg muscles, or shift weight during the experiment. Repeat the experiment using the second subject.

When you have completed the experiments, construct graphs to show the results obtained for each subject. Three readings should be shown: systolic pressure, diastolic pressure, and heart rate (see illustrations on pages 53 and 54).

Note that the first illustration shows only slight changes in blood pressure and heart rate, while in the second illustration the heart rate increases markedly the longer the subject stands quietly. This is not unusual. In many subjects both the diastolic and systolic pressures remain fairly constant but the heart rate increases rapidly. In one instance a seventeen-year-old girl in good health showed a heart rate of 65 beats per minute while lying down. But during the quiet standing phase, her heart rate accelerated to 200 beats per minute.

Compare the results of the tests you have just completed for the two subjects. Are the results similar or are there slight or major differences? If the differences are significant, how do you account for them?

OVERCOMING GRAVITATIONAL FORCE

When someone is standing quietly, without moving his or her body, the force of gravity causes blood to collect in the lower part of the body. Because of the lack of bodily movement, the gravitational force is not overcome by skeletal muscles forcing the blood upward. When the return of the blood to the heart is decreased, this causes a lowering of blood pressure, in particular in the systolic phase. To maintain blood pressure, the heart rate

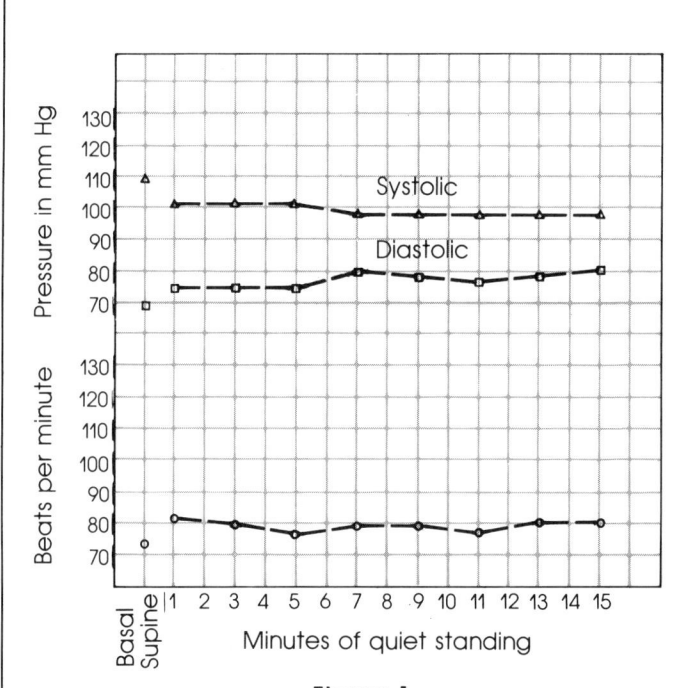

**Figure 1
Blood pressure
and heart rate
during quiet standing**

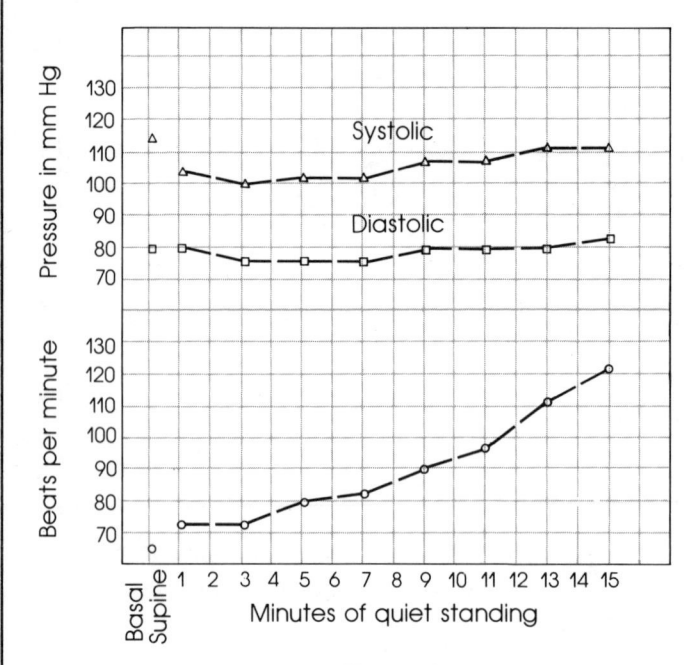

Figure 2
Blood pressure and heart rate during quiet standing

increases. This is an example of physiological feedback. However, in cases where the blood pressure and heartbeat both remain fairly constant (as seen in the first illustration), it is reasonable to assume that the subject's vasoconstriction mechanism is maintaining the blood pressure.

Note: For some subjects the stress of quiet standing may cause dizziness or even fainting before the fifteen-minute period is completed. This can happen in subjects who appear to be in excellent health. As soon as a subject indicates that he or she feels dizzy, the subject should be urged to sit or lie down. Also, subjects should not be asked to take part in the experiment if they have missed breakfast or lunch or are overtired.

Did the age or sex of the two subjects selected for your tests make any difference in the results? If so, explain why. Did the stress of quiet standing cause dizziness or a feeling that fainting might occur if the time period were extended?

PROJECT 7:
Recovering from exercise

Equipment and materials:
sphygomomanometer, stethoscope, metronome, notebook, pencils, graph paper, stopwatch

In this demonstration project you will also need an assistant to help you record data. Use two subjects, one a smoker and one a nonsmoker. Your subjects should be young adults in good health (the smoker should not be a student). Use the nonsmoker for the first experiment. Before the subject begins exercising, ask him or her to lie down for a few minutes. Then take the subject's blood pressure and heart rate, recording your results in your notebook.

Now begin the exercise test. Ask the subject to step up on a chair and back down again to the beat of a metronome. One suggested rate is 63 steps per minute for a period of three minutes. Then ask the subject to return to a resting position. Begin recording the subject's blood pressure and heart rate simultaneously until they have returned to normal or remained constant for at least three minutes. Chart the results on a graph.

Does the recovery from exercise show a more standard pattern than the results you obtained from the standing-still experiment? Or are the variations more unusual? How long did it take for the nonsmoking subject's blood pressure and heart rate to return to normal? If your subject is a healthy fellow student who is active in athletics, his or her recovery probably did not take very long (note: in the first illustration the recovery to normal blood pressure and heart rate was complete within five minutes). If your subject is not an athlete and doesn't exercise regularly, recovery probably took longer. What other factors should be taken into account in assessing the results of this test?

Repeat the experiment using the subject who smokes. Before you begin the test, find out how long the subject has been smoking and how often he or she smokes (cigarettes, pipe, or cigars). If the subject smokes cigarettes, note the brand and whether or not it is a filtered cigarette. When you have completed the test, chart the results on a graph. How does the smoker's recovery from exercise differ from the results you obtained from the nonsmoker? If the difference is significant, how do you account for it? What apparent effect does smoking have on the body's cardiovascular system?

PROJECT 8:
Respiration and heart rate

Equipment and materials:
nomogram, spirometer, recorder or kymograph with ac-

cessories for recording respiratory movements, stopwatch, notebok, pencil

In calculating total lung capacity, four volumes of air must be measured: tidal air volume, inspiratory reserve volume, expiratory reserve volume, and residual air volume. The tidal air volume is the amount of air which is inhaled during normal breathing. The amount of air that can be inhaled in addition to the amount of air inhaled during normal breathing is the inspiratory reserve volume. Similarly, the expiratory reserve volume is the amount of air that can be exhaled in addition to the air normally exhaled during quiet breathing. The air that remains in the lungs after the expiratory reserve volume has been exhaled is the residual air volume.

The maximum amount of air that can be brought into the lungs and forcefully exhaled is known as the *vital capacity*. There are many factors that govern a person's vital capacity, including size and physical condition. Gender is another governing factor. The vital capacity of a man is greater than that of a woman of the same body size. Many diseases can also affect the vital capacity, in particular pneumonia, emphysema, changes in blood vessels as a result of heart disease, and the presence of tumors in the thoracic cavity.

CHANGES IN RATE AND DEPTH OF BREATHING

When you are breathing normally, you are usually unconscious of this rhythmical body process. You inhale and exhale without any particular conscious effort. The changes in rate and depth of breathing are usually well regulated according to the needs of your body. The dominant factors in regulating breathing are the amount of carbon dioxide in the blood, the amount of oxygen in the blood, and the blood's pH factor (the measure of its acidity or alkalinity). These factors can change according to body activity, causing a change in respiratory movements and heart rate when appropriate.

Select a subject for this experiment. Interview the subject to find out about his or her lifestyle, including eating and drinking habits, the amount and forms of exercise or athletic activity, age, weight, and if the subject smokes. Record the information in your notebook.

Now determine the surface area of the subject's body, using a nomogram (see illustration on page 59). Hold a straightedge so that it intersects the left vertical line of the nomogram at the point where the subject's height is indicated and the right vertical line where the subject's weight is indicated. The point at which the straightedge intersects the middle line will show the surface area of the subject's body expressed in square meters. Use this information to determine your subject's vital capacity in liters. For women the vital capacity is approximately 2 liters/square meter of body surface area; for men it is approximately 2.5 liters/square meter of body surface area. This will give you the estimated value of your subject's vital capacity.

To find out how closely your estimate compares with the subject's actual vital capacity, you will need to use a spirometer. This is a water-filled container into which air is exhaled. The volume of air exhaled is automatically recorded on a dial (see photograph on page 60). First clean and dry the mouthpiece of the spirometer with soap and water or alcohol. Then set the needle of the spirometer at zero.

Ask your subject to stand erect and inhale as deeply as possible. Place the mouthpiece of the spirometer in your subject's mouth. Ask the subject to hold his nostrils closed and exhale as much air into the spirometer as possible without bending over. As the subject exhales, the inner chamber of the spirometer rises, with the needle on the dial recording the amount of air in the chamber.

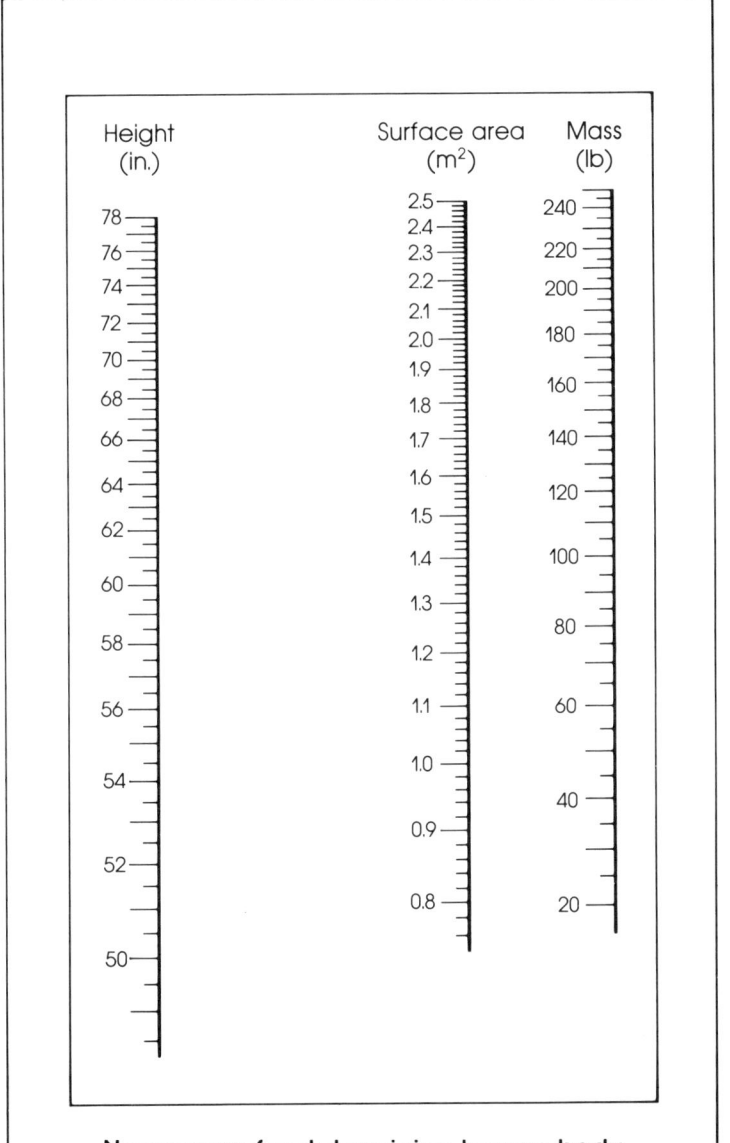

Nomogram for determining human body surface area

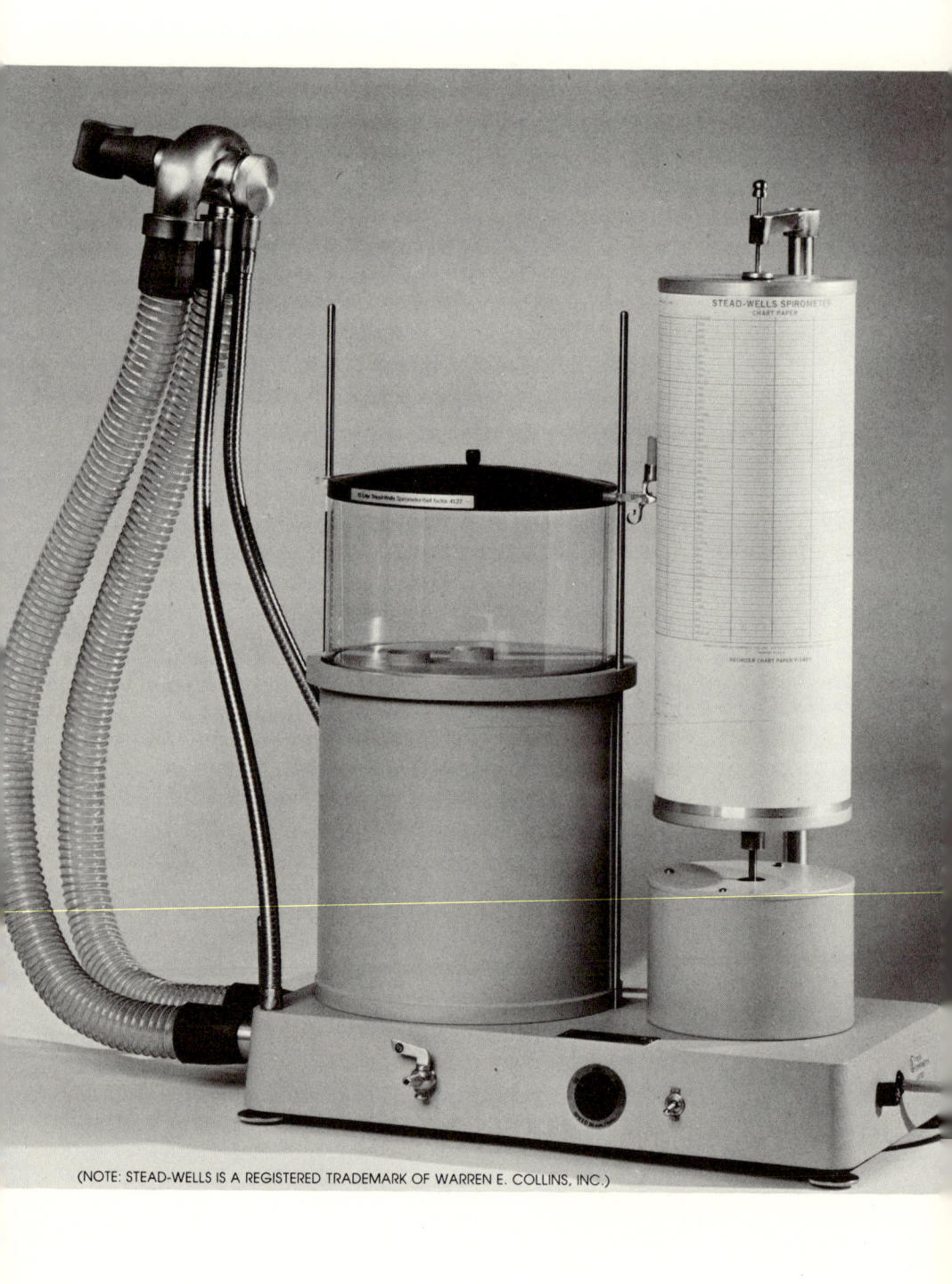

(NOTE: STEAD-WELLS IS A REGISTERED TRADEMARK OF WARREN E. COLLINS, INC.)

When the test is completed and the mouthpiece removed from the subject, the spirometer chamber returns to its original position. Do not push it down or water will be forced out of the chamber. Reset the needle on the spirometer at zero and repeat the test two more times. Calculate and record the average of your readings.

RECORDING RESPIRATORY MOVEMENTS

Either a recorder or a kymograph with the appropriate accessories may be used to record your subject's respiratory movements (see illustrations). The following discussion will be confined to use of the recorder with the following accessories: an event/time marker module, a tambour module, and a pneumograph. Note: The capillary pens on the two modules should be adjusted so that they are horizontal and parallel to one another. The ink flow should be started in both pens.

The pneumograph is an expandable piece of tubing that fits around the subject's chest. Each time the subject breathes, the pressure inside the pneumograph changes, causing a deflection of the tambour's capillary pen or stylus. The small chain on one end of the pneumograph should be fastened on a hook at the other end to hold the pneumograph in place on the subject's chest. The pneumograph should be fastened at the level where the greatest chest movement occurs during each inhalation. Fasten it tightly enough to the subject's chest so that it won't slip down, but not too tightly.

Note the section of rubber tubing on the pneumograph. This contains a glass or metal T-connection. On

A SPIROMETER
AND KYMOGRAPH

one arm there is a short piece of rubber tubing with an attached clamp. Be sure to release the clamp before you connect the pneumograph to the tambour; then tighten it securely just before you begin recording. The tubing on the other arm of the T-connection should be attached to the projecting metal tube on the side of the tambour module on the recorder. Make sure the connection is airtight. If necessary, secure a wire around the rubber tubing. Once the connection is made, tighten the clamp on the pneumograph tubing. Each time your subject inhales and exhales, the capillary pen or stylus on the tambour should move. Be sure to keep the pneumograph in the same position on the subject's chest throughout the experiment.

Ask the subject to face away from the recorder. Record six or eight normal inhalations and exhalations, at the same time adjusting the speed of the chart paper so that the peaks and waves are about 5 mm apart. As each series of recordings is made, write on the chart paper what is being recorded. Ask your subject to stand erect and inhale as deeply as possible. With his nostrils closed, the subject should then exhale as much air as possible. This records the vital capacity you measured earlier with the spirometer (see illustration on page 63).

Now divide the vital capacity reading you obtained from the spirometer test (ml) by the height of the vital capacity obtained from the recorder (mm). Your answer will indicate the number of milliliters of air represented by a height of 1 mm on the recording. Here's an example: if the vital capacity obtained from the spirometer reading was 4,000 ml and the height of the vital capacity reading on the recorder was 40 mm, this shows that a vertical distance of 1 mm on the recording represents 100 ml. 4,000 ml/40 mm = 100 ml/mm.

On your chart paper and data sheet, record the number of milliliters of air indicated by each milliliter on the recording. The chart paper should be labeled to indi-

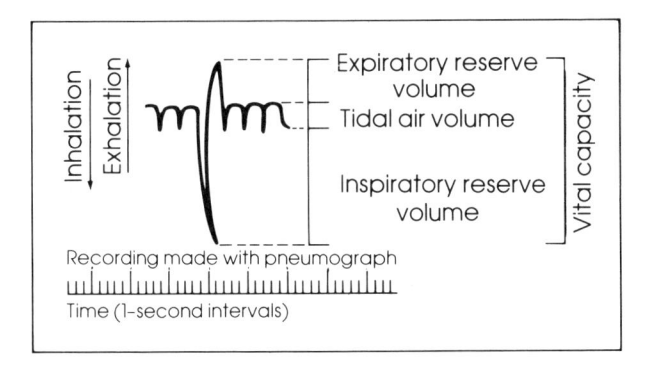

**Recording of
respiratory movements**

cate the portions of vital capacity recorded that consist of inspiratory reserve volume, tidal air, and expiratory reserve volume. After all of your recordings have been completed, calculate the quantity of air comprising each of these portions.

THE OXYGEN/ CARBON DIOXIDE EXCHANGE

You will now test the relative effects of an increase in inhaled carbon dioxide and a decrease in inhaled oxygen on the respiratory rate and depth and heartbeat. Record six or eight of the subject's normal inhalations. Give the subject a small plastic bag containing about a liter of air and ask him to place it tightly over his face. Ask your subject to rebreathe the air from the bag until you note a change in respiratory rate and depth. Take the subject's pulse and record the heart rate in your notebook. Then remove the plastic bag from his face and allow his respiratory movements to return to normal.

For the second phase of this experiment, use the same plastic bag but this time add a small quantity of soda lime. This absorbs carbon dioxide. Repeat the test for the same period of time as before. As the test proceeds, the oxygen levels will decrease; however, the carbon dioxide levels in the air being breathed will not increase. What difference does this make in the results of the test? How do your results compare with the previous test?

Continue the series of experiments by making recordings while the subject is (1) speaking, (2) swallowing, and (3) coughing. Note the effect these actions have on the rate and depth of breathing.

To record the effects of recovery from exercise, disconnect the pneumograph from the tambour, but leave it around the subject's chest. Ask the subject to exercise vigorously for two or three minutes. Suggestions: Ask the subject to run in place, or step on or off a chair. Immediately following the exercise, quickly reconnect the pneumograph to the tambour and record the subject's breathing and heart rate during his recovery period. Note the time necessary for the subject's respiratory rate and heartbeat to return to normal.

Now test the effects of hyperventilation and hypoventilation. Ask your subject to sit down and hold his breath as long as he can (hypoventilation). Record how long he is able to do this. Take the subject's pulse when he resumes breathing, noting the effect hypoventilation has had on his heart rate. Now ask your subject to hyperventilate, that is, to inhale deeply and exhale quickly about ten times. As soon as he has completed this part of the test, take his pulse and record the effect of hyperventilation on his heart rate. Once more ask the subject to hold his breath for as long as he can and note how long he is able to do so. Is there any difference in the length of time he is able to hold his breath from the first time you measured it? Is there any change in the effect it has had on his heart rate?

MEASURING RESPIRATORY MINUTE VOLUME

In the final phase of this experiment, measure your subject's respiratory minute volume. This is the total amount of air taken into the lungs in a period of one minute. You calculate the volume by multiplying the volume of air inhaled in one breath—the tidal volume—by the number of breaths per minute. You have already taken recordings from which you can calculate the volume of air inhaled. The event/time marker will show the time represented by a given segment of the recording. This is the information you need to calculate the minute volume.

Using previous recordings, calculate the minute volume during quiet breathing and record the volume in your notebook. Then calculate and record the minute volume immediately following exercise. After you have determined these volumes, calculate and record in your notebook the following information:

1. The percent increase in the minute volume following exercise.
2. The percent increase in the volume of each inhalation following exercise.
3. The percent increase in breathing rate following exercise.
4. The increase in heart rate following exercise.

Write a summary of the results of this project in which you answer the following questions:

Which has more effect on changing rate and depth of breathing and heart rate: increasing levels of carbon dioxide or decreasing levels of oxygen?

Why does hyperventilation result in a change in the length of time a subject can hold his breath? What effect does hyperventilation have on heart rate? How does this relate to the effects of air pollution on heart rate?

How did your subject's *measured* vital capacity compare with his *estimated* vital capacity? How can you account for the fact that a person's vital capacity may be different from the estimate for his or her body size?

Which showed the greater change following exercise—the quantity of air inhaled in each breath or the breathing rate? Explain the effects of exercise on heart rate.

PROJECT 9:
The effect of emotional stress on the heart

Equipment and materials:
sphygmomanometer, stethoscope, stopwatch, notebook, pencil

Imagine you are an athlete preparing for an important game or a student about to take an examination. You are likely to be nervous and worried about the result. In situations like these, your emotions can get the upper hand and cause stress. This can have a direct effect on your blood pressure and heart rate.

A wide range of emotions can directly affect the functioning of the heart. Emotions such as fear, rage, anger, resentment, frustration, and anxiety, for example, have been shown to stimulate the nerve centers in the brain. These, in turn, cause the pituitary gland to stimulate the thyroid and adrenal glands, among others, to produce hormones that contribute to an increase in pulse rate, blood pressure, and other actions of the heart. The volume of blood pumped from the heart may be increased in response to the need for more oxygen for the body's tissues and organs. Intensely felt emotions may also cause irregularities in the rhythm of the heartbeat.

Under normal conditions a certain amount of stress is both necessary and healthy, from the moment of birth onward. A newly born baby, for instance, needs to feel enough stress to take the first life-giving breath. In order to do well in their school work, students must feel enough stress or anxiety to want to perform at their best. The same is true for athletes as they prepare to begin a game or competition. They need to feel tension or stress so they can concentrate their abilities to perform at their best.

For this project, select two subjects in situations in which a certain amount of stress is anticipated. One subject could be a leading athlete about to play a major game. The other could be a fellow student about to take an important exam. The day before the event, take each subject's blood pressure and pulse rate and record the data in your notebook. Repeat these tests on the day of the event, one hour and one half-hour before the event takes place. Immediately after the event, record the subject's blood pressure and pulse rate. Then repeat the tests one hour after the event. Make a graph of the results obtained from each subject.

Which of the two subjects showed the greatest increase in blood pressure one half-hour before the event? Which of the two subjects' blood pressure returned to normal more quickly after the event had been completed? To what do you attribute the difference in results?

In preparing the subjects for the series of blood pressure and pulse rate readings, which subject appeared calmer? What do you know about their personalities and lifestyles that may account for the difference in results?

PROJECT 10:
Controlling responses to emotional stress

Equipment and materials:
sphygmomanometer, biofeedback machine, stethoscope, stopwatch, notebook, pencil, graph paper

A great deal of research has been devoted to finding ways to reduce stress in human beings, especially in those who have a high blood pressure condition. Dr. Herbert Benson of Harvard Medical School, author of *The Relaxation Response*,[*] believes that most people have the ability to overcome stress by using the techniques he has developed to cause the body to relax. Unlike most reactions to stress, which are involuntary, the relaxation response is voluntary. A conscious mental effort is made to control physiological responses, such as blood pressure, heart rate, and blood flow or volume. This technique is similar to those employed by practitioners of yoga, Zen

---

[*]Herbert Benson, with Miriam Z. Klipper, *The Relaxation Response*. New York: Morrow, 1976.

Buddhism, and transcendental meditation. First developed in the Eastern part of the world, these techniques have recently become familiar to people in many Western nations, including the United States.

In his research Dr. Benson conducted many experiments using Eastern relaxation techniques as well as techniques that he had devised. Many of the volunteers had high blood pressures. By developing the relaxation response, they were able to lower their blood pressures so long as they practiced relaxation methods twice a day. When some of the subjects stopped using relaxation techniques, however, their blood pressures rose to hypertensive levels within four weeks.

Dr. Benson's method involves the use of a biofeedback technique. This is similar to other relaxation techniques in that a mental effort is used to lower blood pressure and change other physiological responses. The important difference in biofeedback, however, is the use of electronic devices, such as the biofeedback machine.

The biofeedback machine is set up to measure a particular physiological response, such as blood pressure. In indicating the level of blood pressure, the biofeedback machine emits a series of signals. The subject responds by making a conscious mental effort, such as thinking peaceful thoughts, to lower his blood pressure and thereby change the signals. The machine responds by feeding back the results of the subject's efforts. When the efforts are successful, the signals change to indicate a drop in tension and blood pressure (see photograph on page 70).

According to researchers, the success of the biofeedback technique may depend to a significant degree on the subject's personality. Type A and Type B personalities are often used as examples. The Type A personality is very time-conscious, competitive, impatient,

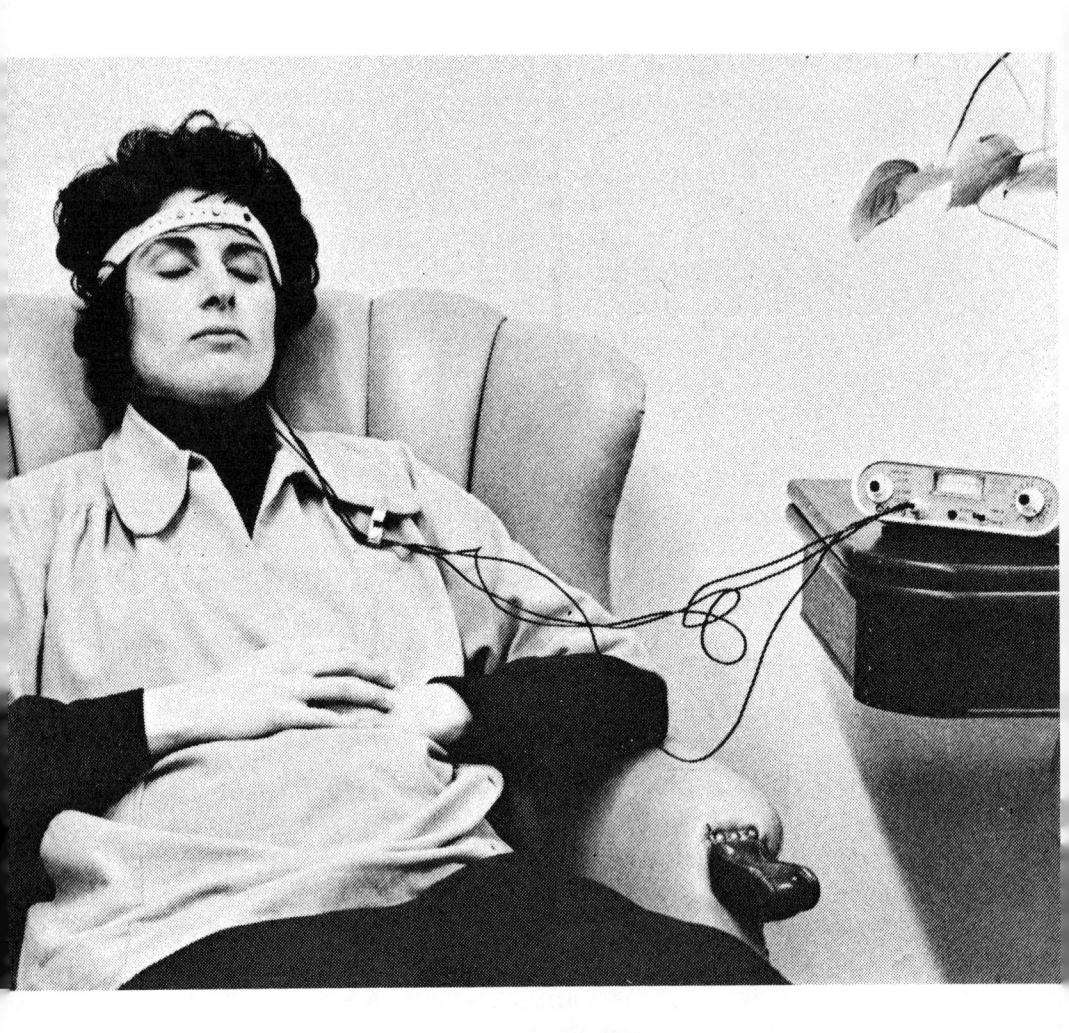

A PATIENT USING A
BIOFEEDBACK MACHINE

hostile, and often short-tempered. The Type B personality tends to put off work and decisions or not to worry about them. He or she appears to be under no time pressure. Type B might also be described as a "low-keyed" or an "easygoing" individual. Type B personalities are less likely to be hypertensive than Type A.

For this project select two subjects who have some of the qualities of the Type A personality. One subject should be a person or fellow student with no known history of hypertension. The other person should be a person known to be hypertensive or who is being treated for high blood pressure (perhaps some family member or relative would agree to be your subject). Subjects should be as similar in lifestyle and body structure as possible.

In each case, the subject sits comfortably in a chair for a few minutes. Take his or her blood pressure and pulse rate and record the data in your notebook. Then attach the electrodes from the biofeedback machine to the subject's forehead to measure the muscle tension produced by his or her blood pressure level. Ask the subject to make a conscious effort to relax by thinking peaceful thoughts. Note any changes this produces in the signals emitted by the biofeedback machine. The subject should continue to make a conscious effort to relax until a reduction in blood pressure occurs. Continue the biofeedback technique for a period of fifteen minutes. Then take the subject's blood pressure and pulse rate and record the data in your notebook.

Did the biofeedback technique have an effect on the blood pressure of the first subject, the one with no known history of hypertension? What results did you obtain using this technique on the second subject, the one with a high blood pressure problem? After concluding this project, what is your opinion of the biofeedback technique? Do you believe that a person can exert mental control over physiological responses, such as blood pressure and heart rate?

PROJECT 11:
The effect of stimulants and depressants on heart rate

Equipment and materials:
microscope, daphnia (live specimens), microscope slides, stopwatch, droppers, cotton fibers, 10^{-5} chlorpromazine, 10^{-5} d-amphetamine sulfate, 0.5% ethanol, coffee, carbonated beverages, other stimulants and depressants, graph paper, notebook, pencil

The live specimen used in this project is the daphnia, a small aquatic animal sometimes incorrectly called a "water flea." The daphnia is a relative of crayfish and shrimp and is commonly found in ponds and streams. Daphnia are also grown in large quantities at fish hatcheries and aquarium supply houses as food for fish. One of the most unusual features of this tiny specimen is its transparency. With the aid of a microscope you will be able to observe the functioning of its internal organs, including the heart (see photograph on page 73).

Using a dropper, select two daphnia specimens from a culture jar and place them on a slide. Try to remove as much water as possible from the slide, but leave enough to keep the organism alive. You may want to restrict the movement of the animals before you proceed with the experiment. This can be done by placing a few cotton fibers under the cover slip. When you place the slide under the microscope at low power, you should be able to see the hearts beating very rapidly. Note and record the rate of heartbeat under normal conditions by counting the number of beats per minute for three successive minutes. Be careful not to confuse the heartbeat with the rhythmic beating of the animals' antennae.

Record all three rates. (You may want another student to assist you by serving as timekeeper.) Note: it may help to reduce the amount of light so you will have a clearer view of the beating heart. Reducing the light also prevents a temperature rise that might kill the animal.

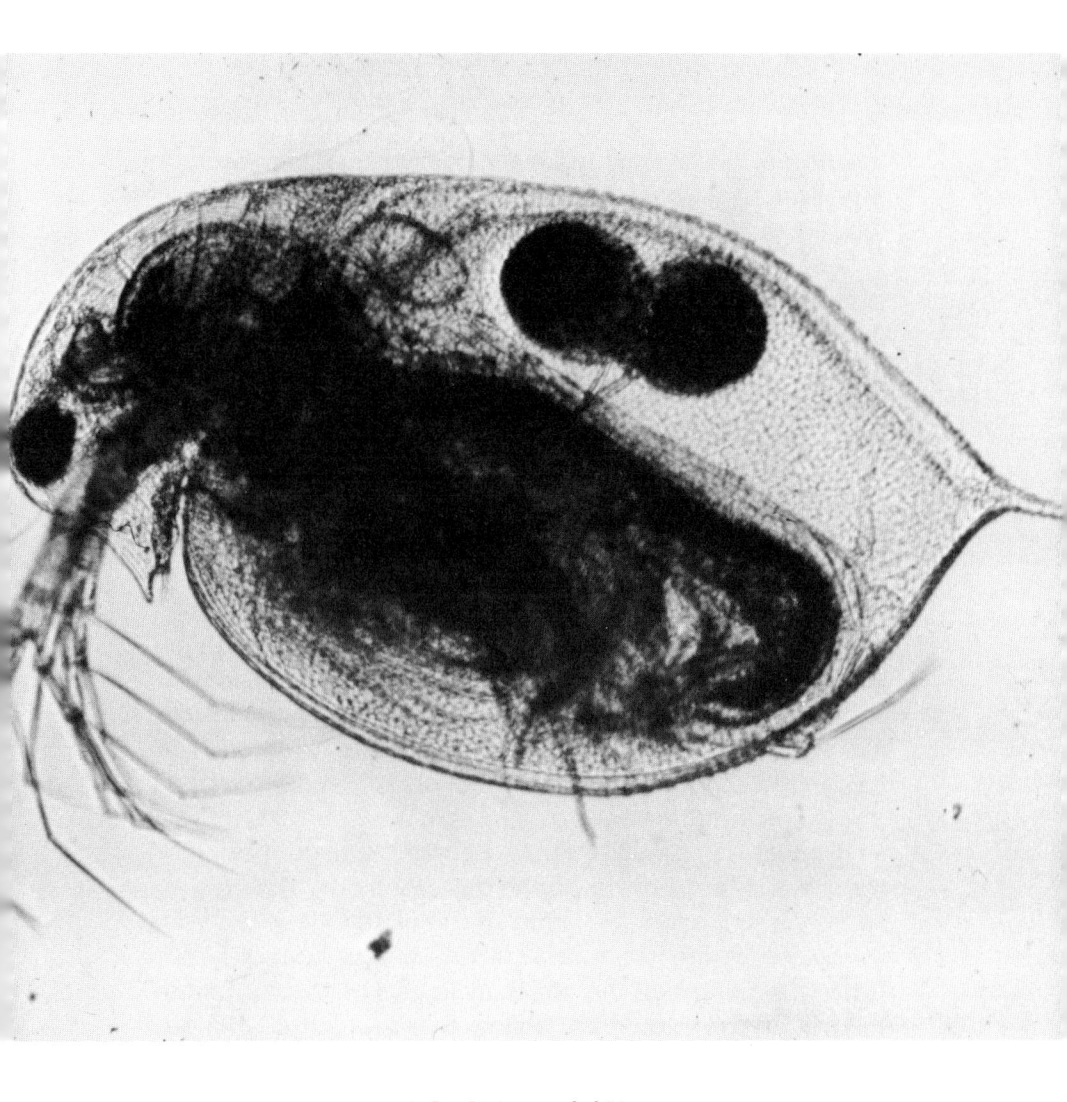

A DAPHNIA AS SEEN
THROUGH A MICROSCOPE

Place a drop of chlorpromazine solution on the slide and note the reaction of the daphnia. Take three readings of the heart rate as before, counting the number of beats per minute for three successive minutes. Record the data in your notebook. Now rinse the dropper thoroughly and use it to put the daphnia back in the jar.

Select another daphnia and place it on a clean slide, removing as much water as possible. Note the normal heart rate as before and record the information in your notebook. Now put a drop of d-amphetamine sulfate solution on the daphnia and observe the animal's reaction. Record the heartbeat rates as before.

Repeat the above procedures using the alcohol solution. For each set of figures (the heart rate determined over a three-minute period), calculate the average heart rate.

Continue the experiment using solutions containing coffee, carbonated beverages, and other stimulants and depressants and record the results in your notebook. Construct two charts, one showing the variations in the normal heart rate of the specimens used in the experiment, the other showing the variations when depressants and stimulants were used.

Which of the first three chemicals used had the greatest effect on the daphnia's heartbeat? How great was the variation in normal heart rate? How do you account for the differences, if any, in the normal heart rate? Comment on the results obtained using other stimulants and depressants, noting those which produced the greatest changes in heart rate.

PROJECT 12:
The effect of exercise on heart muscles

Equipment and materials:
bandage or cloth to use as tourniquet, sphygmomanometer, stethoscope, stopwatch, notebook, pencil

Select two subjects for this project. One should be an athlete or someone who exercises regularly, such as a jogger. The other subject should be someone who rarely exercises. Begin the experiment by observing the venous flow of both subjects in a test similar to that used by William Harvey, the English physician and anatomist who discovered blood circulation. Apply a tight bandage or tourniquet around the arm above the elbow of the athletic subject. Note: This tourniquet should not be left in place for more than two minutes. Ask the subject to clench his or her fist. You will notice that the veins of the hand and forearm swell. There will probably also be localized swellings at intervals on the veins.

Using one finger, press down firmly on a part of the vein close to the hand. Use another finger to press the blood along the vein away from the hand. Press the blood beyond the next swelling. Does this cause the vein to empty? Now remove the second finger and note the reaction. Does the vein fill up?

Now use your second finger to press the blood toward the hand, noting the result. Remove the first finger and note from which end the vein starts refilling. Lastly, with your finger moving down over a vein, try to force the blood toward the hand. Repeat these procedures, using the nonathletic subject.

Note and record all these observations in your notebook, explaining what happened and why. Were there any significant differences in the results obtained from each subject? What does this experiment tell you about the factors responsible for the return of blood to the heart?

For the next phase of the project you will need two students to assist you in taking the pulse rate, respiration rate, and the systolic and diastolic blood pressures of each subject. Ask the first subject, the athlete, to sit quietly for five minutes. Take his or her "resting" pulse rate, blood pressure, and respiration rate (one minute). Now ask the subject to perform physical work or exercise, such as the "standing-running" exercise. A rate of two steps per second for one minute is suggested. Then take the pulse rate, blood pressure, and respiration rate. Wait two minutes and then ask the subject to repeat the exercise for one minute. Record the pulse rate, blood pressure, and respiration rate.

Wait two minutes and then ask the subject to repeat the exercise, once again noting and recording the pulse rate, blood pressure, and respiration rate. Now let the subject rest for five minutes and then take his or her pulse rate, blood pressure, and respiration rate. Repeat at five-minute intervals until pulse rate, blood pressure, and respiration rate have returned to normal. Repeat the above procedures, using the second subject, the nonathlete.

Analyze all of the data obtained from the two subjects and comment on the differences in the results. What does this reveal to you about the importance of exercise in strengthening heart muscles and heart function?

5
CONSTRUCTION PROJECTS

Whatever science fair or science competition you plan to participate in, there are certain rules you must follow as carefully as possible. These rules will include guidelines and restrictions concerning the construction project you will need for your exhibit. The construction project or display unit must be built within certain size and weight dimensions. It must also meet the required safety standards, such as in the use of electricity and electrically-powered equipment. If you plan to use living animals in your exhibit, your project should meet the standards specified in *Regulations for Experiments with Animals* of the National Science Fair-International. These guidelines were created by the National Society for Medical Research and later amended by committees of the Animal Care Panel and Institute of Laboratory Animal Resources.

**PROJECTS IN WHICH
ANIMALS WILL BE USED**

The *Regulations* state that these five guidelines should be followed:

1. The basic aim of scientific studies that involve animals is to achieve an understanding of life, and to advance our knowledge of life processes. Such studies lead to a respect for life.
2. A qualified adult supervisor must assume primary responsibility for the purposes and conditions of any experiment that involves living animals.
3. No experiment should be undertaken that involves anesthetic drugs, surgical procedures, pathogenic organisms, toxicological products, carcinogens, or radiation unless a trained biological scientist, physician, dentist, or veterinarian directly supervises.
4. Any experiment must be performed with the animal under appropriate anesthesia if pain is involved.
5. The comfort of the animal used in any study shall be a prime concern of the student investigator. Gentle handling, proper feeding and provision of appropriate sanitary quarters shall at all times be strictly observed. Any experiment in nutritional deficiency may proceed only to the point where symptoms of the deficiency appear. Appropriate measures shall then be taken to correct the deficiency, if feasible.

All of these guidelines should be discussed with your instructor before you proceed with any project in which live animals will be used.

**SELECTION OF
CONSTRUCTION MATERIALS**

The first thing to keep in mind in selecting materials to use in your construction project is that they must suit your purposes. You have a wide range of materials to select from, but whatever you choose should be sturdy and durable. If your exhibit is successful in a state competition, for example, you may want to enter regional or national competitions. Sturdy and durable materials, however, do not have to be heavy and cumbersome. There are many lightweight materials that will be adequate for your needs and at the same time make transporting the exhibit to competitions as convenient and inexpensive as possible. Any heavy equipment, of course, should be well supported so there will be no danger of its tipping over.

Pay close attention to the design of the exhibit, avoiding an inclination to either overbuild or underbuild. The overall design should highlight and reinforce the results of your project. Take advantage of your instructor's knowledge and experience in working out the details of the design and construction. Even though you may have worked out a design that meets your needs and pleases your sense of aesthetics, be flexible. Be willing to make changes that others believe would improve the presentation.

THE SCIENCE PROJECT AND THE EXHIBIT

Your exhibit will highlight the results of your science project, but it is only one of several important elements in your presentation. Your efforts in gathering materials, researching related experiments, consultations with your instructor and other professionals, all the details about your experiments, results, and conclusions will be contained in your research paper. This is the most important document in your presentation. Showing the results of your project as clearly and as dramatically as possible is evidence of how well the project was conceived and completed. It is of prime importance for the impression it will make on the judges at the science competition.

You might wish to use a three-sided display. This can be set up to stand by itself on one long table. You can then use two smaller tables at either side of the exhibit as well as one long table in front, if that suits your purpose. If you choose to use a three-sided exhibit, the central portion could contain the title of the project and a summary statement of the research design.

On the side panels, or wings, you could highlight the purpose and procedures (on the left panel) and your results and conclusions (on the right panel). Graphs, diagrams, photos, drawings, and other visual materials could be interspersed where appropriate to reinforce your statements. On the smaller side tables and the long table in front of your exhibit, you could display samples of the equipment and materials used as well as your scientific paper.

In selecting a sturdy material for the three panels, you might want to consider ¼-inch (0.6-cm) plywood or 1-inch (2.5-cm) styrofoam framed in wood or some other material that would be sturdy but not too heavy. The three panels would have to be hinged or taped together (depending on the type of material used) and secured to the tabletop. The next step would be to paint the paneling, selecting a color that will provide a good background for the lettering you will use for the project title and the titles of the other sections (purpose, procedure, results, conclusions, etc.). You might want to cut out the lettering from construction paper, use individual plastic letters, or use stencils and paint the lettering onto the panels.

If you plan to use drawings, it is a good idea to outline the drawings in a light pencil first until you get exactly what you want. Then use a marking pen (black or some other color) for the final rendering. If you want to make a large drawing from a small one, use a projector to blow up the drawing onto a large sheet of white paper or posterboard. Then trace the enlarged drawing in pencil and make your final rendering with a marking pen.

Photos that are clear and sharp can also be used to enliven your exhibit. If you've taken a series of photos to show the steps taken in the project, select the best photos and have enlargements made to 5" x 7" or 8" x 10" size. Remember that the photo alone will not tell the story. You'll need to write captions for each photo, describing what the photo illustrates. The captions should be written in large letters or produced by a local printer, so they will be easy to read.

PROJECT 1:
How the human heart functions

Design and construct a display which shows how the human heart functions in maintaining the body.

Suggestions: Show the differences and similarities in the arterial and venous circulation of the blood. Highlight the importance of respiration in regulating the oxygen–carbon dioxide exchange. How do heart rate and blood volume affect the body's circulatory system? What role does the heart play in regulating blood pressure?

PROJECT 2:
High blood pressure

Make a display that illustrates the causes of high blood pressure and shows how this endangers heart function.

Suggestions: Use drawings, photographs, and X-ray photos to show the effects of arteriosclerosis in obstructing blood flow, resulting in elevated blood pressure. Also illustrate how obstruction of blood flow causes ischemia, or loss of oxygen, which can damage body tissues. Show other causes of high blood pressure and how they endanger heart function.

PROJECT 3:
The dangers of smoking

Make a display that illustrates how cigarette smoke inhaled into the lungs decreases the oxygen supply, causes a narrowing of blood vessels, and makes the heart work harder.

Suggestions: Show the results of experiments in which both smokers and nonsmokers were used as subjects. Highlight differences in blood pressure, heart rate, and respiratory rate at rest and after exercise. Use photographs, drawings, and X-ray photos to show the effect of smoking over a long period. Use the same materials to show how stopping smoking improves heart rate, blood pressure, and respiratory rate as well as the health of the lungs.

PROJECT 4:
Exercise and the heart

Make a display to show the effect of exercise in strengthening heart muscle, heart function, and blood circulation.

Suggestions: Show the results of experiments in which both athletes and nonathletes were used in exercise tests. Data should include differences in pulse rates, blood pressure, and respiratory rates. If practicable, test athletic subjects before the season begins for their sport, at mid-season, and when the season has ended. For one of your nonathletic subjects, if possible include someone who has just started a jogging or running program to strengthen the heart and improve his or her overall physical condition. Test this subject at two-week intervals for a period of six weeks and document any changes in heart rate, blood pressure, and respiratory rate, before and after exercise tests.

PROJECT 5:
Breathing

Use a working model to demonstrate the process of breathing. The model should show the movements of both the diaphragm and chest wall. Show how the blood absorbs oxygen in the lungs and is circulated to the rest of the body. Show how carbon dioxide and other waste products are exchanged and eliminated when the blood returns to the heart through the body's venous system and then is pumped into the lungs.

Suggestions: The model's chest should be transparent so the action of the rib cage and diaphragm in forcing air out of the lungs can be shown, as well as how the heart functions in blood circulation and the oxygen and carbon dioxide exchange. Based on experiments you have conducted, show the results of hyperventilation and hypoventilation on heart rate, blood pressure, and respiratory rate before and after exercise.

PROJECT 6:
Blood vessels

Construct a device or model to illustrate the relation of arteries, capillaries, and veins to one another.

Suggestions: You may want to use a full-length drawing of an adult human as well as photographs and X-ray photos for close-ups of blood circulation in the heart, lungs, and other parts of the body. Blood circulation within the major blood vessels and the vessels of the heart itself can be demonstrated by the use of X-ray photos taken after a radiopaque tracer has been injected into the blood. You may be able to obtain these photos from a local radiologist, a doctor who specializes in taking and analyzing X-ray photos. Explain how the direction of blood flow is controlled. Explain the differences in blood volume, pulse rate, and respiration rate between a normal person and a person with some form of heart disease or high blood pressure.

PROJECT 7:
The structure of the mammalian heart

Demonstrate the structure and function of the mammalian heart by using an untrimmed pig, beef, or sheep heart obtainable from a local butcher or slaughterhouse.

Suggestions: You may want to use a plastic model of a human heart as well as an untrimmed pig, beef, or sheep heart for this exhibit. Explain the similarities and differences in control of heart function, pointing out factors that make the human heart more susceptible to mental and physical stress.

PROJECT 8:
How the heart beats

Construct a display in which the heart of a frog has been removed and placed in a dish of Ringer's solution. The beating of the heart outside the body demonstrates the ability of cardiac muscle to contract without receiving a nervous stimulus from outside the heart.

Suggestions: Explain the action of the pacemaker in causing the heart of an amphibian to contract without receiving a nervous stimulus. Show how this is also true in the case of humans and other mammals. Describe and illustrate how the heart gives off and receives electrical impulses. Use sample electrocardiograms to illustrate the electrical action of the heart when it is functioning normally and when it is functioning abnormally because of heart disease, high blood pressure, or other health problems.

PROJECT 9:
Age and heart rate

Make a chart showing the relationship of age to heart rate. Use subjects from different age groups, including young children and the elderly, with data taken while subjects are resting and after exercise.

Suggestions: Plan to use a blowup of the chart as the central panel in an exhibit. In addition to showing how age affects heart rate, also highlight the differences in blood pressure and respiratory rate when subjects are at rest and after exercise. Further explore this area by showing the effect of heart rate on the circulatory system in normal, healthy subjects and in subjects with health problems.

PROJECT 10:
The heart in space

Prepare a display that shows how astronauts can be protected from changes in forces that affect the efficient operation of the heart and circulatory system.

Suggestions: Write to the National Aeronautics and Space Administration (NASA) for information, photographs, and other illustrative material. Ask specifically for material about experiments on astronauts (men and women) in weightless or gravity-free environments at the Space Center in Houston and during space missions. Illustrate the effects of a gravity-free environment on heart function, blood circulation, and respiratory rate. Also show the effects of space missions on these functions in astronauts after they have returned to earth. Explain any problems that may have occurred. Show how heart function responds to and depends on gravity in a normal, healthy adult human at rest, during exercise, and after exercise. Use subjects of different age and gender. Construct a chart to show the results of your experiments.

6

WRITING A SCIENTIFIC REPORT

Your scientific report will be the most important element in any science fair or competition you enter. Through your scientific report you reveal how well you understand the project, how thoroughly and carefully you have conducted it, and how meaningful and understandable it will be not only to you but to your peers, your instructor, and those judging the competition.

Before you begin to outline and then write the report, you should review the results of all the steps taken in the project. This should include:

1. The plan and design of the project.
2. Notes from your review of research by others (books, magazine articles, etc.) that relates to your project.
3. Lists of materials and procedures.
4. All recorded observations.
5. Data organized into tables, charts, diagrams, and graphs.
6. Photos, drawings, and other visual records such as recorder or kymograph readings, electrocardiograms, nomograms, and X-ray photos obtained from professional sources to help illus-

trate or reinforce your results and conclusions.
7. Conclusions or summaries which are interpretations of your results.

THE ELEMENTS OF A SCIENTIFIC REPORT

The first elements to appear will be the title page, acknowledgments, and table of contents. These will be followed by your statement of purpose, abstract, review of the literature, materials and methods, results and conclusions. The last element is your bibliography, a listing of sources (books, magazines, and other periodicals) that you have referred to in your scientific report.

The only information to appear on the title page will be the title of the project, your name, class in school, name and location of school, and the date your scientific report was completed. For the next page, the acknowledgments, you should write a brief acknowledgment citing those who have assisted you with your project. This should include those who gave you advice and guidance and those who made materials, equipment, and facilities available to you.

The table of contents is a listing of the sections of your report and the pages on which they appear. There should be seven major sections: statement of purpose, abstract, review of literature, materials and methods of procedure, results, conclusions, and bibliography. Your statement of purpose should be a brief resume of what you intend to show as the result of your project. This can be done in a few sentences and should include any hypotheses you expect the project to prove or illustrate.

Probably the most difficult section to write in your scientific report is the abstract. This is a brief and highly condensed summary of your project and should contain the essence of your purpose, procedure, results, and conclusions. The abstract should not exceed 300 words in length. You will probably write a better abstract if you do not write it until you have completed all the other sections of your scientific report. Before you begin writing, review several examples of well-written abstracts in award-winning scientific reports and projects.

The body of your scientific report should begin with your review of the literature. The notes you have taken while reading books, magazines, and other periodicals about projects that relate to yours will form the basis for this section. This should be a brief section. It will be interesting to the reader to know what sources you have consulted before beginning your project; but what you have actually done in your project is of the greatest interest to readers, especially those who will be judging your project. As you move on to other sections of your report, however, you may want to make reference occasionally to some of these sources, where appropriate. Wherever specific references are made to the results of someone else's research, you must be sure to acknowledge the source. This can be done by giving the last name of the author and the date of publication in parentheses immediately following the reference, or by the use of a footnote.

Now we come to the "nuts and bolts" of your project, the section on materials and methods of procedure. This should be a careful and thorough account of the materials and equipment used in each step, the tests performed, and the data recorded. In the results section, which follows, you should include any graphs, charts, diagrams, and other illustrative material to show how the results were obtained and analyzed. Captions should be written for each of the illustrations used, briefly explaining the purpose and results.

In your conclusions section you will be interpreting and evaluating the results of your project. Like your abstract, this section should be given a great deal of thought before you begin to put words to paper. Read over everything that you have already written in the other sections (except the abstract, which you will be writing last). Then make your analysis of what the results appear to indicate. Do the results justify or prove your hypotheses? Are the results conclusive? Now that the project has been completed, be forthright in pointing out the weaknesses as well as the strengths of the project design. If you feel it is appropriate, express your opinions on how the project could be improved. It may also be appropriate to discuss any questions that the project has left unanswered and which you believe could be explored in another project.

The final section of your scientific report or research paper is the bibliography. This is the list of books, magazine articles, pamphlets, and other written sources you have used in researching your project and writing your report. These sources should be listed alphabetically by author. Use the following format for books: last name of author, first name and middle initial, title of book, where published, name of publisher, and year of publication. For articles in journals or magazines: last name of author, first name and middle initial, title of article, name of publication, volume number or date, and page numbers of the article. Here are examples:

(book) Noble, Arthur W. *The Stress Factors in Blood Pressure*. New York: Belvedere Press, 1984.

(magazine) Burrough, Robert E. "Heart Function in Space Shuttle Missions." *Human Physiology Journal* 57: 80–86.

7

PREPARING FOR SCIENCE COMPETITIONS

Each science fair has its own requirements and limitations, but no matter what competition you may be entering, you will be judged on four essential criteria: personal knowledge, originality, presentation, and scientific content. One of the most important reasons for any competition is to discover scientific potential. Your project should clearly show not only a scientific contribution in its own right but a contribution to your educational development. In other words, your project should offer proof that you have learned certain scientific principles and how to demonstrate them. It should also demonstrate your ability to use scientific methods effectively.

Any project that exactly duplicates another project performed in the past lacks the essential criterion of originality. But even if you base parts of your project on well-known experiments, your project can still be original if you ask questions that have not been asked before. In other words, you can use a basic research approach and then add your own personal input to make the project your own.

One of the most important elements in your presentation is your construction project or exhibit. A good presentation, however, does not have to be complex or heavily detailed in order to demonstrate your skills as a scientist. In fact, if you plan an exhibit design that is simple in concept, you will probably have a greater impact. All the essential elements must be there, carefully and logically organized. The construction itself should show good use of available materials. The message should be clear and well supported by the facts and results you present.

The scientific content of your project should demonstrate your ability to use scientific methods effectively. Your research should be thorough and so should your experiments, observations, and analysis of results. The project should also clearly indicate its importance as a scientific problem concerned with society's welfare.

8

PRIZES, SCHOLARSHIPS, GRANTS AND OTHER AWARDS

The following list highlights some of the national competitions available to high school students but does not include state or regional competitions. Your instructor may have information about these and other competitions you may want to enter.

EARTHWATCH

Earthwatch offers Field Research Internships for students and Teacher Fellowships. Grants are available toward the costs of participating on any of the over eighty projects that Earthwatch sponsors worldwide. The disciplines covered are varied, in field locations nationwide, as well as in thirty foreign countries. Most of the projects are conducted during the summer.

All students between the ages of sixteen and twenty-three are eligible to apply for these funds, pending availability. Students are requested to complete the usual expedition application, specifying which projects they are interested in, and send this with a letter outlining their financial needs to the Education Department at Earthwatch. Each applicant will be notified within one month of receipt of his or her application. For applications and more information write to Daryl W. Eaton, Manager of Admissions, Earthwatch, 10 Juniper Road, Box 127, Belmont, Massachusetts 02178.

INTERNATIONAL SCIENCE AND ENGINEERING FAIR

The International Science and Engineering Fair, held annually in different regions of the U.S., offers more than 450 awards sponsored by General Motors Corporation and about forty-five special awards sponsored by other organizations, including the American Medical Association, the American Society for Microbiology, and the Weizmann Institute of Science. The competition is open to students from the ninth to twelfth grades. Two winners are selected from each of the affiliated fairs held at local, state, and regional levels. The costs for entry fee, transportation, meals, and housing for students and accompanying adults are provided by the affiliated fairs.

Awards from General Motors include first place ($250), second place ($175), third place ($100), and fourth place ($50) in each of twelve categories. Categories include behavioral and social sciences, biochemistry, botany, chemistry, earth and space sciences, engineering, environmental sciences, mathematics and computers, medicine and health, microbiology, physics, and zoology. The special awards from sponsoring organizations include cash awards; expense-paid trips to scientific and engineering installations and national conventions; oceanographic cruises; summer jobs; plaques, medals, books, magazine subscriptions, and certificates. For applications and more information write to Science Service, 1719 N Street NW, Washington, D.C. 20036.

JACKSON LABORATORY
SUMMER STUDENT PROGRAM

This program is sponsored by Jackson Laboratory, Bar Harbor, Maine. Applicants must be in their junior year of secondary school, at least fifteen years of age by the date the summer program starts, and have completed at least one course in biology. They must be United States citizens and must not have attended a summer student science training project supported by the National Science Foundation. Scholarships of up to $850 toward the participant fee may be requested by applicants who require financial aid in order to attend the nine-week program. The $850 covers board, room, supplies, and services. Students are required to purchase medical insurance for about $15 and may take advantage of the optional linen service for about $15.

First organized in 1949, this precollege program enables superior secondary school science students to participate in current biomedical research. Each participant works full-time on an independent research project under the supervision of a staff member. Bench work is supplemented by a series of lectures and demonstrations and discussion groups. Students present oral and written reports at the conclusion of the program.

Applications must be submitted by April 1. Candidates are notified by April 30. The program begins in the middle of June. For applications and more information write to the Jackson Laboratory, Summer Student Program, Bar Harbor, Maine 04609.

NATIONAL SCIENCE FOUNDATION
SCIENCE TRAINING PROJECT

The National Science Foundation, an independent agency of the federal government, supports various programs to strengthen education in the sciences, engineering, and mathematics. Each summer the National Science Foundation provides scientific training programs for about 3,000 high school students of high ability. For applications and more information write to Public Information Branch, National Science Foundation, Washington, D.C. 20550.

NSTA/NASA SPACE SHUTTLE STUDENT INVOLVEMENT PROJECT

Sponsored by the National Science Teachers Association (NSTA) and the National Aeronautics and Space Administration (NASA), this program provides an opportunity for secondary school students to propose experiments suitable for possible testing aboard the space shuttle and, where appropriate, for performance by the astronauts. The purpose is to stimulate interest in science and technology by directly involving students in a space research program. The program is open to students in grades 9 through 12 in all U.S. public, private, parochial, and overseas schools, including U.S. civil and military overseas establishments, Puerto Rico, Guam, and the outlying territories.

Students may propose an experiment suitable for testing aboard the space shuttle by conforming to the rules of the competition. It is not intended that an experiment be constructed or performed by the student. However it is imperative that proposals deal with concepts which utilize one or more of the unique features of the space shuttle, such as a microgravity environment, operation above earth's atmosphere, or a broad view of the earth's surface. The proposal text may not exceed 1,000 words.

Up to twenty students in each of the designated ten geographic regions will be selected as regional winners. All regional winners and their teachers/advisors will be awarded an expense-paid trip to a special Space Shuttle Symposium held at a NASA research center in the spring. From the regional winners, up to ten national winners will be selected. All national winners and their teachers/advisors will be invited to a National Space Shuttle Symposium, expenses paid, where they will receive awards for themselves and their schools. All proposals of national winners will be considered for selection by NASA for possible flight on a future space shuttle mission. For applications and more information, write to National Science Teachers Association, NSTA/NASA Space Shuttle Student Involvement Project, 1742 Connecticut Avenue, NW, Washington, D.C. 20009.

WESTINGHOUSE SCIENCE TALENT SEARCH

Sponored by Westinghouse Electric Corporation and the Westinghouse Educational Foundation, Science Talent Search is administered by Science Service. Approximately $90,000 is awarded in scholarships to forty winners (1984 awards included one $12,000 scholarship, two $10,000, three $7,500, four $5,000, and thirty awards of $500 each). The competition is open to high school seniors in public, private, or parochial schools in the U.S. and Puerto Rico who are expected to complete college entrance qualifications by October 1 of the following year. The forty winners are invited to attend the five-day Science Talent Institute in Washington, D.C., all expenses paid. Winners must bring a project exhibit to the Institute which will be displayed to the public. It need not be the project submitted in the competition.

In addition to the forty top winners, there are 300 winners of Honorable Mention awards, who will be brought to the attention of all colleges, universities, and technical schools in the U.S. Hundreds of students will automatically receive recommendations and other assistance toward a college education in schools within states holding State Science Talent Searches.

Teachers or other school officials must request entry materials for the outstanding science and mathematics students of the school. A completed entry consists of a project report of about 1,000 words which presents evidence of research ability in science or engineering; a personal data blank filled in by the student, teachers, and principal; national test scores and high school transcript.

Judging is based primarily on the student's report on an independent research project in the physical sciences, behavioral and social sciences, engineering, mathematics, or biological sciences, (excluding live vertebrate experimentation). Entries must be received no later than midnight, December 15. For applications and more information write to Science Service, 1719 N Street NW, Washington, D.C. 20036.

APPENDIX

The following is a partial list of suppliers of special equipment, animal specimens, organs, and other needs for the projects presented in this book. Where a supplier specializes in certain equipment and materials, this is indicated in parentheses.

AO Scientific Instruments, Buffalo, NY 14240

Beckman Instruments, Inc., Bioresearch Marketing, P.O. Box 3100, Fullerton, CA 92634

Carolina Biological Supply Co., Burlington, NC 27215

Cole-Parmer Instrument Co., 7425 N. Oak Park Avenue, Chicago, IL 60648

Eastman Kodak Company, Dept. 412-L, Rochester, NY 14650 (laboratory chemicals)

Frey Scientific Company, 905 Hickory Lane, Mansfield, OH 44905

Graphic Instruments Division, Gulton Industries, Inc., East Greenwich, RI 02818

Harvard Apparatus Company, 22 Pleasant Street, South Natick, MA 01760

Lab Products, Inc., 255 West Spring Valley Avenue, Maywood, NJ 07607

Olympus Corporation of America, 4 Nevada Drive, New Hyde Park, NY 11042

Research Products Div., Miles Laboratories, P.O. Box 2000, Elkhart, IN 46515

Sargent-Welch Scientific Company, 7300 North Linder Avenue, P.O. Box 1026, Skokie, IL 60077

Unitron Instruments, Inc., 175 Express Street, Plainview, NY 11803

Carl Zeiss, Inc., One Zeiss Drive, Thornwood, NY 10594 (optical instruments)

INDEX

Accuracy, 11
Age and heart rate, 85
Angina pectoris, 50
Animal experiment guidelines, 77–78
Animal heartbeats, 3
Aorta, 14, 15, 36, 37
Arrhythmias, 32
Arteries, 13, 14, 17, 20
Arterioles, 14, 50
Atria, 13, 14, 25, 35, 36
Atrioventicular valves, 17, 37

Benson, Herbert, 68, 69
Bibliography, 90
Biofeedback, 69, 71
Blood, oxygen in, 4–5, 6, 13–15, 67
Blood circulation, 2–4, 13–15, 17, 83; respiration and, 37–39
Blood pressure, 13, 37, 67, 68; high, 50–52, 69, 71, 81; lifestyle and, 22–23; measurement of, 17–24
Blood vessels, 2, 13, 15, 83–84
Brachial artery, 20, 22

Brain, 4, 6

Capillaries, 14
Carbon dioxide, 2, 5, 6, 13, 14, 57, 64–65. *See also* Oxygen-carbon dioxide exchange
Chemicals, effects on heart, 42–44, 72–74
Chorda tendinae, 15, 37
Circulatory process, 13–15
Competitions, 7, 77, 87, 91–98
Construction projects, 77–85
Controlled experiments, 10
Coronary vessels, 15

Demonstration projects, 35–76
Dependent variables, 10
Depressants, effects on heart rate, 72–74
Diaphragm, 5, 6
Diastolic pressure, 17, 19, 20, 22
Dizziness, 55
Drugs, effects on heart, 44–50

Earthwatch, 93–94
Eastern relaxation techniques, 68–69
Electrical activity of heart, 24–33
Electrocardiogram, 25, 28–33
Electrocardiograph, 25–33
Emotional stress, 1, 4, 66–71
Emphysema, 57
Environment, reactions to, 24
Error, sources of, 9
Exercise, 4, 50, 82; effect on heart muscles, 74–76; electrocardiograms and, 32; recovery from, 23, 55–56
Exhibits, 77–85, 91–92
Experimental control, 9

Fairs, 7, 77, 87, 91–92
Feedback control, 24
Food additives, effects on heart, 43, 72, 74
Frenulum, 48

Galvanometer, 25
Gravity, 52–55
Guidelines for animal experiments, 77–78

Harvey, William, 3, 75
Heart: blood flow and, 17–24; effects of chemicals and drugs on, 42–50, 72–74; electrical activity of, 24–33; emotional stress and, 1, 4, 66–71; smoking and, 32–33; sounds, 23; in space, 85; structure and function, 13–15, 35–37, 81, 84
Heart attack, 50
Heart disease, 25, 50
Heart rate, 2–4, 13, 14, 17, 24, 51, 52, 84, 85; age and, 85; effects of stimulants and depressants on, 72–74;

Heart rate (*continued*) respiration and, 56–66
High blood pressure, 50–52, 69, 71, 81
Hormones, 67
Hypertension. *See* High blood pressure
Hyperventilation, 65
Hypothesis, 9
Hypoventilation, 65

Independent variables, 10
Infantile paralysis, 5
International Science and Engineering Fair, 94

Jackson Laboratory Summer Student Program, 95

Korotkov's sounds, 19–20, 22

Lifestyle and blood pressure, 22–23
Lungs, 4–6, 37–38, 57

Mammalian heart, 35–37, 84
Materials, exhibit, 78–81
Methods, scientific, 9
Mitral valves, 17, 36
Muscles, heart, 5, 14, 15; exercise and, 74–76

National Science Foundation Science Training Project, 95–96
National Society for Medical Research, 77
Nervous system, 3, 4, 5–6
Nomogram, 58
NSTA/NASA Space Shuttle Student Involvement Project, 96–97

Observation projects, 13–33
Oscillograph, 25

Overventilation, 37–38
Oxygen, 2; in blood, 4–5, 6, 13–15, 67; consumption, and pollution, 39–42
Oxygen-carbon dioxide exchange, 13, 37–39, 57, 64–65

Pacemaker, 14
Papillary muscles, 15, 37
Pericardium, 35
Peripheral resistance, 50
PH factor of blood, 57–58
Physiological feedback, 55
Pituitary gland, 67
Pneumograph, 61, 62
Pneumonia, 57
Poliomyelitis, 5
Pollution and oxygen consumption, 39–42
Pulmonary artery, 15, 36
Pulmonary veins, 4, 5, 13, 14, 15, 36
Pulse pressure, 19
P wave, 25, 30, 32

Q wave, 25, 30, 32

Recovery from exercise, 23, 55–56
Regulations for Experiments with Animals, 77
Relaxation, 68–71
Repetition, 9
Reports, scientific, 87–90
Research, 9
Respiration, 4–6, 82; blood circulation and, 37–39; changes in rate and depth of, 57–61; heart rate and, 56–66; oxygen-carbon dioxide exchange, 13, 37–39, 57, 64–65
Respiratory minute volume, 65–66

Respiratory movement, 61–64
Ribs, 5, 6
R wave, 25, 30, 32

Scholarships, 93–98
Scientific reports, 87–90
Semilunar valve, 36, 37
Sinus node, 32
Smoking, 32–33, 55–56, 82
Sounds, heart, 19–20, 22, 23
Space, heart in, 85
Sphygmomanometer, 19–24
Standing still, heart's response to, 51–52
Stethoscope, 19–24
Stimulants, effects on heart rate, 72–74
Stress, 1, 4, 66–71
Stroke, 50
Stroke volume, 50, 51
S wave, 25, 30, 32
Systolic pressure, 17, 19, 20, 22, 51

Thyroid gland, 67
Timing, 10–11
Trial and error, 9
Tricuspid valves, 17
T wave, 25, 30, 32
Type A personality, 69, 71
Type B personality, 69, 71

Vagus nerve, 14, 39
Valsalva's experiment, 38–39
Variables, 10
Vasoconstriction, 50
Veins, 13
Vena cavae, 5 13, 15, 36
Venous system, 14
Ventricles, 13, 14, 17, 35, 51
Venules, 14
Vital capacity, 57, 58, 62

Westinghouse Science Talent Search, 97–98